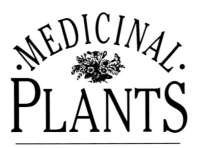

·MEDICINAL·
PLANTS

·MEDICINAL·
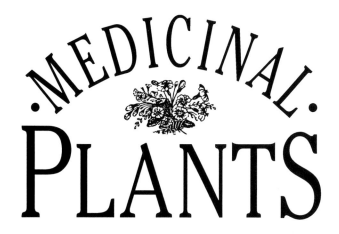
PLANTS

AN ILLUSTRATED GUIDE
TO MORE THAN
180 HERBAL PLANTS
— GEORGE GRAVES —

Foreword by Dr A. Hollman

BRACKEN BOOKS
LONDON

Medicinal Plants

The illustrations in this book are reproduced from the original
plates in *Hortus Medicus*, published 1834, and from those in
Woodville's *Medical Botany* published in 1790.

This edition first published in 1996 by Bracken Books, an
imprint of Random House UK Ltd, Random House, 20 Vauxhall
Bridge Road, London SW1V 2SA

ISBN 1 85170 527 9

Printed and bound in Singapore

PUBLISHER'S NOTE
Many of the plants described in this book are poisonous.
While a number are still used in homeopathic remedies on no
account should they be experimented with without first
consulting a professional opinion. The publishers cannot
accept responsibility for any illness arising from the misuse of
these plants.

LIST OF PLATES
[Numbers shown are page numbers]

FOREWORD

George Graves F.L.S. (1754–1839) was a colourer and artist and also an editor. He produced the third edition of William Curtis' *Flora Londinensis*, the first edition of which contained many plates coloured by his father, and he compiled several other works of natural history between 1811 and 1834. They comprise: *British Ornithology* in three volumes "with a coloured representation of every known species of British Birds"; *Monograph of the British Grasses*; *Ovarium Brittanicum* "a delineation of the eggs of birds native in Great Britain"; *The Naturalist's Pocket Book*, and the *Naturalist's Journal and Miscellany*. In spite of this large output he was often in debt especially over the *Flora*, which Sir Joseph Hooker said was due to incredible mismanagement. But he and his wife (a Curtis) brought up a family of eight and did well by them. His co-author Dr J D Morries was a distinguished Edinburgh physician and author of papers on the chemistry of plant products.

The present work appeared in 1834 under the title *Hortus Medicus* or figures and descriptions of the more important plants used in medicine, or possessed of poisonous qualities; with their medicinal properties, chemical analysis, &c. &c. by George Graves, the chemical and medical departments by John Davie Morries, M.D. It is dedicated to the junior members and students of the medical profession. By containing both botanical and medical descriptions of plants it is in fact a herbal and follows in a long tradition started by Dioscorides in A.D. 100 and exemplified in Britain by John Gerard's fine herbal of 1597. However after about 1700 botany and medicine began to produce their own separate literature with floras and pharmacopeias respectively so this is a late example of the genre.

Medical plants are well described in the earliest medical writings of 3000 B.C. and their use must go back well before recorded history. We have just no idea how these medicines were originally discovered except that it must have taken many centuries of self experimentation to learn for example that mandrake root was a powerful analgesic and hypnotic. It was community-based knowledge that gradually led to the identification of the 20 or so plants that yield major drugs used in medical practice today. Sometimes the active principle comes unaltered from the plant – as with morphine from the opium poppy. At other times development of the modern drug has owed everything to intervention by medical science, for example the anti-cancer drug vincristine derived from Madagascar periwinkle. But a great majority of the plants which were held by common usage to be useful medically have turned out to have no therapeutic value. Thus we have the paradox that whilst medicinal plants have given us drugs of great value which no laboratory could have made, it has also produced many hundreds of unproven remedies and some of these are still prescribed by herbalists. It is interesting in this light to survey some of the plants in this book.

The purple Foxglove was being used in the treatment of heart failure (anasarca and hydrothorax) and it is still irreplaceable in the treatment of abnormal cardiac rhythms (palpitation) and some cases of heart failure. Treating heart failure remained a big problem until synthetic diuretics were invented and in Graves' time the excess fluid was removed by violent purging – he mentions especially the spirting cucumber – or by the now obsolete diuretics such as common broom and officinal squill. The family *Solanaceae* has always commanded medical attention and henbane is praised as a valuable narcotic. It contains hyoscine which is the standard pre-operative medication used worldwide today and is also good in sea sickness. Thornapple was used then in asthma and later it and henbane became of great value in the treatment of Parkinson's disease. Deadly nightshade is mentioned for pain relief but the use of its alkaloid atropine for eye disease and heart attacks was yet to come. Meadow saffron, was well known in medicine B.C. and its active principle colchicine still holds a useful place along with synthetic drugs in the treatment of gout. Graves discusses what its mode of action might be and remarkably for the time states that it increases the quantity of uric acid in the urine. Peruvian bark from species of *Cinchona* had a good reputation in intermittent and remittent fevers, that is to say in malaria and the active principle quinine which had just been isolated is preferred, he says, to the whole bark. Modern anti-malarials have not displaced quinine which is still of value. Until recently ipecacuanha, another South American plant, was invaluable in amoebic dysentery but the only modern use referred to is that as an emetic in cases of poisoning. Willow bark is recommended for fevers though oddly not for rheumatism and the newly discovered "vegetable principle" salicin was the basis for the later synthesis of aspirin. Finally, among these botanical drugs which have stood the test of time we find a good description of the alkaloids morphine and codeine which had by then been isolated from the opium poppy.

Other useful but less important medicines which are mentioned include several remedies for constipation such as rhubarb, castor oil and senna, whilst the value of dill for colic in babies is stressed. Liquorice and cardamom helped to make the ubiquitous bottle of medicine more palatable but sometimes medicines were deliberately made nasty especially for neurotic patients and nothing excelled the nauseous flavour of asafoetida. Some plants which are poisonous are also valuable in therapy, but the book, as the original title shows, deliberately includes quite a number which are only poisonous. The reason for this lies in the need to tell poisonous plants from those used in medicine, or equally importantly for food. Good examples of this are the fungus amanita, fool's parsley, and the hemlock water dropwort, a deadly poison which gets mistaken for edible roots. Culinary plants are well described. Allspice, clove, nutmeg, pepper and cinnamon are mentioned and the housewife is also told about olive oil, sugar, oranges, how to make bread and the removal of stains with oxalic acid. She can also read about homely remedies such as arnica for bruises, balm tea, aniseed, sorrel and castor oil and learn that no remedy is more efficacious for slight febrile affections than Dover's powder.

The book is in fact a compendium of many sorts of information about the plant world and is by no means confined just to the plants which the physician and apothecary would be using. The length of some irrelevant sections such as how to process sugar cane indicates poor editorial judgement and there seems to be no logical arrangement in the book at all. The botanical descriptions are well done and are comprehensive with clear accounts not only of the plant itself, but also of its habitat. The plates too, both of Graves and Woodville are scientifically accurate and artistically prepared.

When thinking of new medicinal plants it is interesting to realise that several first class modern plant based drugs had not been discovered when this book was written, even though the plants as such were known. Some have been mentioned already and others include: curare, the South American arrow poison used in anaesthesia, Intal for asthma, amiodarone and quinidine for cardiac arrhythmias, cocaine as a local anaesthetic, physostigmine and pilocarpine for glaucoma, podophyllin derivatives and rosy periwinkle extracts for malignancies, and aspirin. This is an optimistic thought for the future.

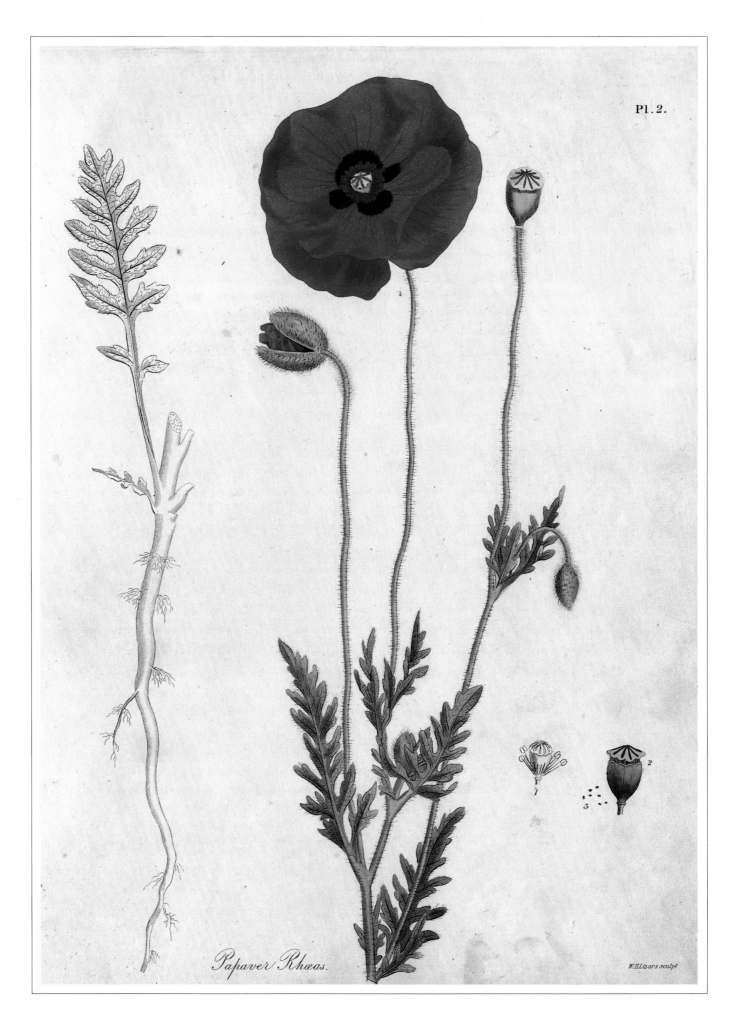

Papaver Rhœas.

Pl. 2.

W.H.Lizars sculpt

8   SMOOTH ROUND-HEADED POPPY; FIG.1, THE GERMEN WITH A FEW STAMENS; FIG.2,
RIPE CAPSULE; FIG.3, SEEDS.

SMOOTH ROUND-HEADED POPPY

Papaver rhœas

Class and Order, POLYANDRIA MONOGYNIA. NAT. ORD. PAPAVERACEÆ.
Gen. Char. *Calix* of two leaves; *Petals* four; *Stigma* sessile, radiated; *Capsule* one-celled, opening with pores beneath the persistent stigma.

ROOT annual, simple; stalk from one to two feet high or more, upright, branched, hairy; flower-stalk upright, each supporting one flower, having the hairs projecting horizontally; calix of two leaves, membranous at the edge, deciduous, hairy, the hairs inclining towards the point; corolla large; the alternate petals smaller, and all of them marked with a shining black spot at the base: Seed-vessel shape of an egg cut off at the top, where it is scolloped, and marked with as many raised lines as there are on the stigma, which is persistent and scolloped on the edge.

The *Papaver rhœas* is occasionally administered to children as an anodyne, but it is retained in Pharmaceutic use more for the fine red colour which it communicates to syrup, than for any medicinal virtue it possesses. It is slightly soothing and anodyne, and is classed among those remedies called pectoral. It is used in slight catarrhal affections. The chemical nature of the colouring matter of the petals is rather interesting. The bright red colour which they impart to water is changed to a green by the action of potass, but not by any of the other alkalies. Solutions of the red in the other alkalies or their carbonates are changed to a green by the addition of potass.

PURPLE FOXGLOVE

Digitalis purpurea

Class and Order, DIDYNAMIA ANGIOSPERMIA. NAT. ORD. SCROPHULARÆ, JUSS.
Gen. Char. *Calix* of five unequal segments; *Corolla* campanulate, swollen beneath, with four or five unequal lobes; *Capsule* of two cells; *Seeds* numerous.

ROOT biennial, or occasionally of longer duration, fibrous; stem erect, three to four, or even six feet high, round, leafy, branching covered with a minute pubescence; leaves large, veined, beneath paler, and downy; flowers pendulous, in long spikes, usually all growing from one side, and hanging one over the other, of a full purple outside, the mouth and interior, elegantly marked with rings and specks of a deeper or paler colour. A variety is sometimes to be met with in the wild state, having white, or rather cream-coloured, flowers, which is likewise commonly cultivated in gardens.

The Foxglove is one of the most common, as well as ornamental, of Britain's native plants, abounding in almost every soil and situation, and, from its size and elegance, must command the attention of every one disposed to admire the beauties of Flora. The genus is somewhat extensive; and, as far as yet ascertained, they are endued with the same properties as the common kind, but in greater or lesser degress of intensity.

Its leaves are collected when the plants are coming into flower, and are often purchased by the druggists in a dry state, than which nothing can be more absurd, as they not only lose much of their active properties by being long dried, but likewise are subject to adulteration by the admixture of other leaves, which in a dry state are not likely to be detected by an inexperienced botanist.

Some writers recommend the leaves to be dried by exposure to heat, which renders them less active, as much of their taste and smell is volatile, and liable to be carried off by heat; a preferable method is to gather the plants in dry weather, and suspend them by the roots in a shady place, where they are exposed to a current of air; when the leaves become dry, they should be removed from the stalks, and packed in close-stopped opaque bottles.

Digitalis, whether employed for the purpose of lessening the rapidity of the pulse, and thus diminishing vascular action, or with the view of increasing the activity of the absorbents, or for promoting the secretion of urine, is both a powerful and useful remedy. It is used in inflammatory affections, chiefly of the chest, in palpitation, arising from hypertrophy or increased action, in phrenitis, in anasarca and hydrothorax, in scrofula, in the leucophlegmatic affection following measles, and in mania arising from effusion. Though generally admitted to be useful, Digitalis is a remedy which must be employed with the greatest caution, inasmuch as its effects on different constitutions are not by any means uniform, and as all the preparations with which we are yet acquainted, are liable to variations, which can only be ascertained by trial on the patient. For this reason, it is always proper, even when the patient has become inured to its use, to commence every fresh quantity of either leaves, extract, or tincture, as if the person were not habituated to its effects. In this way many accidents which occur might be avoided, although, from the almost peculiar property of accumulating on the system, they will occasionally take place. The symptoms produced by an over-dose or by accumulation, are nausea, vertigo, depression, great anxiety, dryness of the mouth and throat, confused sight, sometimes coma or convulsions, and rarely syncope. In cases in which convulsions occur, death generally follows at an interval of two days or more. A case is mentioned by Dr Blackall, in which death did not take place for three weeks.

The effects of digitalis, even in more favourable cases, continue for some time,—particularly the slowness of pulse. The treatment generally recommended is the administration of diffusible stimuli, such as ether and ammonia, combined with opium or aromatics. Opium in the form of clyster has also been found useful. Blisters to the epigastrium, and sinapisms to the legs and thighs, are also mentioned.

WAKE-ROBIN OR CUCKOO-PINT

Arum maculatum.

Class and Order, MONŒCIA POLYANDRIA. NAT. ORD. AROIDEÆ.
Gen. Char. *Spathe* of one leaf, convolute at the base; *Perianth* wanting; *Spadix* with germens at the base; *Stamens* sessile near the middle of the spadix, which is naked above; *Berry* of one cell and many seeds.

ROOT perennial, tuberous, growing horizontally, and furnished with numerous single fibres, which grow from every side; leaves large, usually three or four from a root, broadarrow shaped, on long foot-stalks, generally marked with dark purple blotches; fructification enclosed in a large spathe, the edges of which wrap over each other at the bottom, at the top closing, the middle part compressed; the spadix clubshaped, shorter than the sheath, varying in colour from a pale green to a lively purple; below surrounded by the germens, and withering before them: Stamens, filaments very short, thick, of a pale brownish yellow; anthers ovate, generally in pairs, purplish brown, two-celled; the cells obliquely horizontal, opposite, united at their upper ends; germens numerous, surrounding the base of the spadix, of an ovate roundish shape, placed beneath the stamens; stigmas oblique, beaded with little hairs; berries corresponding in number with the germens, scarlet, roundish, of one cavity; seeds two, ascending, alternately inserted into each side of the receptacle, ovato-globose.

This species, abundant in woods, hedge-rows, and banks, is very conspicuous in the spring from its large shining foliage and spathe, and towards the close of summer, when the leaves are decayed, its solitary stalk supporting a cluster of brilliant scarlet berries, is peculiarly striking.

From the violence of its action, the *Arum maculatum* is never employed in medicine. It acts as a drastic purgative in very small doses. Notwithstanding the disagreeable acrid taste of the fresh plant, children have been poisoned by eating it. Orfila quotes from Bulliard the following account:—

"Three woodsman's children ate of the leaves of this plant; they were seized with horrible convulsions. Assistance was procured when too late. The two youngest could not be made to swallow anything. They were bled without success; glysters were given them, but without effect. They died; the one on the twelfth, the other on the sixteenth day. The other child, when seen, was able to swallow, but with difficulty, its tongue being so much swelled as to fill nearly the whole cavity of the mouth; but deglutition became free after blood-letting. Milk, olive oil, warm water, were given in large quantities; diarrhoea came on, which saved the child; it was pretty well restored in a short time, but remained long very lean."

Some of the species in this and other genera of the natural order possess, even in a more remarkable degree than the *Arum maculatum*, the property of causing painful swelling of the tongue. Dr Hooker mentions the case of a gardener who, from merely tasting a bit of the *Caladium seguinum* (Dumb-Cane), was confined to the house for several days by swelling of the tongue, accompanied with excruciating pain. The juice of this last mentioned plant, as well as that of the *Arum ovatum*, is sometimes used by sugar-manufacturers to assist the granulation when

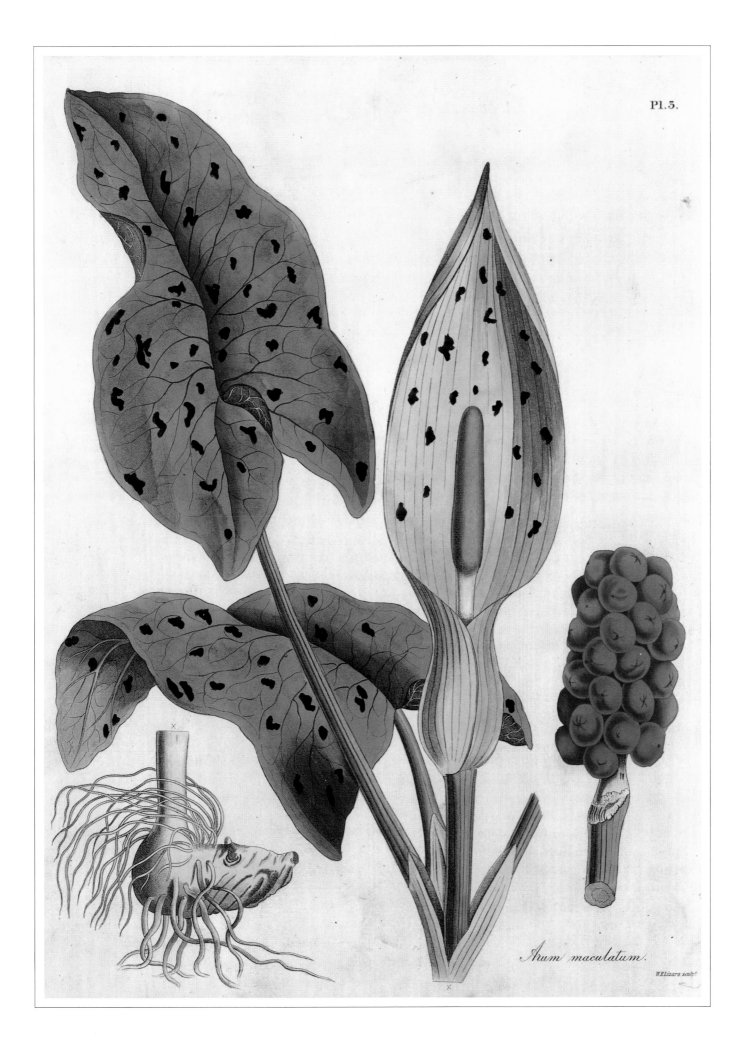

Pl.3.

Arum maculatum.

W.H.Lizars sculp.[?]

WAKE ROBIN OR CUCKOO-PINT

the juice is too viscid. The acrimony of the Arum is entirely destroyed by heat, and though, as has been already observed, a virulent poison when fresh, it becomes not only harmless, but even nutritious when properly prepared. The inhabitants of the Isle of Portland manufacture the fecula and send it to London, where it is sold under the name of Portland Sago. Culture seems to have the power of destroying the acrimony of this genus, and one of the species, the *Arum Colocosia*, is grown as a pot herb.

Cypress powder is prepared from the dried root.

BUCKBEAN

Menyanthes trifoliata

Class and Order, Pentandria Monogynia. Nat. Ord. Gentianeæ..
Gen. Char. *Calix* five cleft; *Corolla* monopetalous, funnel-shaped, hairy within; *Stigma* two-lobed; *Caps.* unilocular.

Root perennial, creeping, long, jointed, and fibrous, flower stems round, simple, procumbent at the base; leaves ovate, smooth, veiny, growing three together on long foot-stalks, which form sheaths at the base, which cover the bottoms of the flower-stalks.

This elegant plant, which is the only known species, is found abundantly throughout Britain, growing in marshy places, and, though formerly held in considerable estimation as a febrifuge, has now fallen almost into disuse.

The *Menyanthes trifoliata* is sometimes prescribed by medical men, in combination with other tonic or febrifuge medicines; but it is much more frequently used as a popular remedy in agues.

Richard speaks highly of its powers as a tonic, and mentions its use in scrofula and rickets. When given in large doses, purging and vomiting are excited, and even a small quantity frequently causes nausea, to prevent which aromatics ought to be combined with it. In Sweden it is sometimes used instead of hops, one part being considered equal to eight of hops. The taste of the whole plant is bitter and disagreeable. The root contains a good deal of fecula, which is used as food in some of the northern parts of Europe.

It appears to me highly probable that the bitter principle is gentianine, and that the purgative and emetic effects are owing to some of the other constituent parts.

THORN-APPLE

Datura stramonium

Class and Order, Pentandria Monogynia. Nat. Ord. Solaneæ.
Gen. Char. *Calix* tubular, deciduous; *Corolla* funnel-shaped, plaited; *Capsule* with four valves.

Root annual, branched; stems from one to four feet in height, or even more, round, smooth, much branched, and spreading; leaves arising from the forking of the stalks and branches, solitary, varying in size, smooth, of a deep-green above, pale beneath, unequally sinuated and toothed, and extending further down the foot-stalk on one side than on the other; flowers single, upright, arising with the leaves from the branching of the stalks, white, funnel-shaped.

The Thorn-apple is often to be met with on dunghills and among rubbish in the vicinity of large towns. It is considered a plant of easy cultivation, growing readily in most soils, and producing a large quantity of seed.

The student will have no difficulty in distinguishing this plant, as we have no other that bears even a distant resemblance to it. Its smell is peculiar, and it possess powerful and very active properties. Of late years Datura has become of considerable interest as a remedy for alleviating the paroxyms of asthma, by smoking it through a tobacco-pipe, a practice imported from the East Indies, where, however, it is not the present species that is used; but the whole genus appears to be possessed of nearly the same properties. That relief may be obtained in certain cases from inhaling the fumes of this plant is without doubt; but that its fumes act differently on different individuals is equally certain. I have found that inhaling the smoke for the space of one minute and a-half, occasioned retching to an uncommon degree, but with this peculiarity, that it was unaccompanied by the straining or exertion usually attendant on vomiting.

Every part of the Thorn-apple, but more especially the seeds, is poisonous; under proper management, however, it becomes a valuable remedy in many diseases. Mania, melancholy, convulsive diseases, such as epilepsy, neuralgic affections, chronic rheumatism, are among the number. In the two last diseases both the exter-

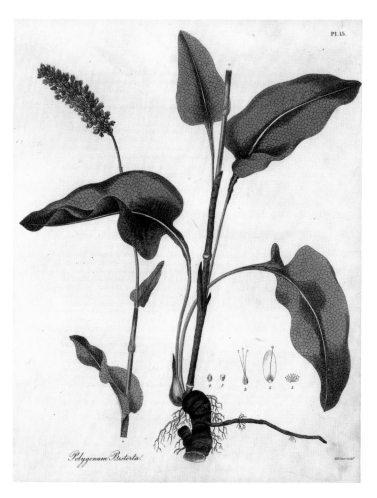

Polygonum Bistorta.

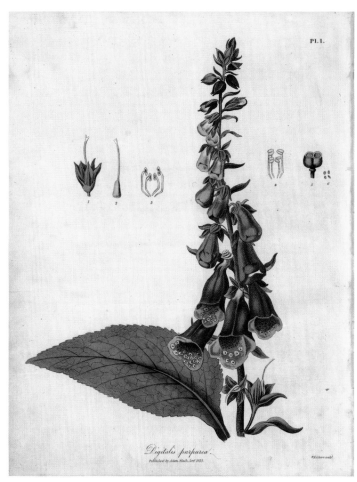

Digitalis purpurea.

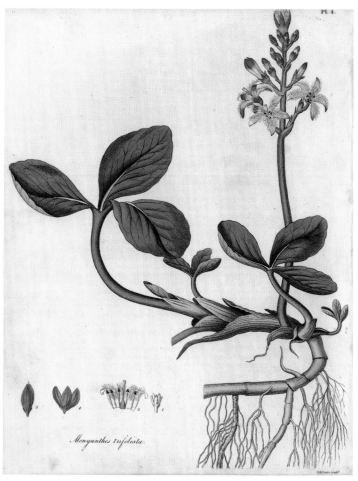

Menyanthes trifoliata.

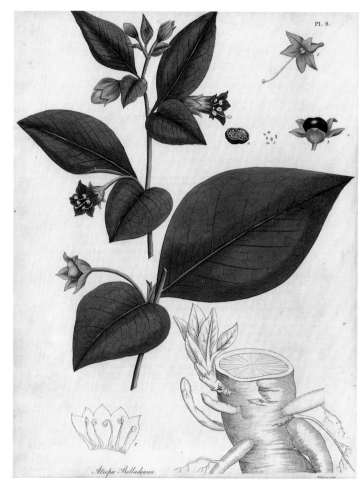

Atropa Belladonna.

TOP LEFT: BISTORT OR SNAKEWEED, TOP RIGHT: PURPLE FOXGLOVE, BOTTOM
LEFT: BUCKBEAN, BOTTOM RIGHT: DEADLY NIGHTSHADE

13

nal and internal use of the remedy is recommended. In hæmorrhoids much benefit has been derived from its application in the form of ointment. Baron Stoerk was the first who used this plant in mania; several Swedish physicians followed his example, and with occasional success. Like the Belladonna, it must be used with caution, both from the violent nature of its effects, and from the uncertain strength of its preparations. The effects produced by a poisonous dose vary with the temperaments of individuals; in general, a kind of intoxication is created, with an inclination to dance, jump, sing, or laugh, (the laugh often sardonic,) then convulsions or paralysis of the limbs, ending in delirium, and that in coma, which may terminate fatally. Paralysis is another affection caused by an over-dose. Sometimes no other symptoms than the intoxication and inclination to muscular motion show themselves, and a sound deep sleep, leaving the person weak and languid, terminates the unpleasant effects.

Owing to the disagreeable and acrid taste of the plant, few accidental cases of poisoning are likely to occur, but there are several on record. Dr Christison mentions, that all recent cases in this country have been accidental, but that in Germany it has been used for the purpose of causing stupefaction, to conceal robbery or some other crime. In India, the *Datura ferox* is used for this purpose, as it acts more directly on the brain than Belladonna. It certainly seems to do so—the delirium which it causes being of a more extravagant nature, and paroxysms of violent madness being not unfrequent.

Richard remarks, that neither this nor the *Atropa* ought to be used when opium can be employed; they are only to be given where opium is contraindicated by some idiosyncrasy, or when it has failed from any other cause. In poisoning by the Stramonium, blood-letting is indicated by the violent determination to the head, and by the circumstance, that after death, the vessels of the brain are generally found turgid. Alkalies, their carbonates, or solution of soap in water, ought to be given if vomiting cannot be caused by emetics. Vinegar is generally recommended as an antidote in cases of vegetable poisoning, but ought never to be exhibited till the stomach be cleared of the poison:—when coma has supervened, perhaps the cold douche might be employed with good effect.

DEADLY NIGHTSHADE
Atropa belladonna

Class and Order, Pentandria Monogynia. Nat. Ord. Solaneæ.
Gen. Char. *Corolla* campanulate; *Stamens* distant; *Berry* with two cavities.

Root perennial, thick, branched, and creeping; stalks several, three or more feet high, upright, rounded; leaves entire, in pairs of unequal sizes; flowers on solitary foot-stalks, drooping, of a livid purple colour; berries at first green, becoming of an intense purple or black when ripe; seeds numerous, brown, irregular in shape, acquiring their brown hue before the berries turn black.

This plant grows in various soils and situations, but appears to abound most in chalky districts; it increases rapidly by its roots and seeds, but, from some circumstance, is found frequently, after flowering, to have the root quite perished before any appearance of decay is observable in the leaves and stems.

The genus Atropa is small, and all the species are said to possess deleterious qualities: the British species is one of the most powerfully narcotic, its unpleasant effects being communicated, both by touch and taste, frequently causing paralysis of the hands from the mere gathering or holding of the plant, and it is this property that constitutes its principal value for medical purposes.

Of all the indigenous poisonous plants with which we are acquainted, not one, perhaps, comes so frequently under the notice of the practitioner as the *Atropa belladonna*. From the tempting appearance of the berries they are often eaten, and as there is nothing nauseous or alarming in the taste, enough are generally taken to produce pretty violent effects. The symptoms of poisoning with Atropa are, dryness and burning heat of the throat and mouth, vertigo, dimness and confusion of sight; dilatation and immobility of pupil; delirium, coma, an eruption resembling that in scarlatina, and occasionally strangury. In Orfila's work on poisons several cases are detailed, of which perhaps the most remarkable is that given by M.E. Gualtier de Glaubry. Of the 150 soldiers who, as he relates, were poisoned by it near Dresden, the greater number were delirious, but the delirium was gay; a great number also lost their voice, and others spoke confusedly; there was also much motion of the hands and fingers; several were blind for some time; and in all, the pupils were dilated.

In Dr Christison's work on poisons, many interesting cases are given, with references to the works containing the full details.

As the stomach becomes nearly insensible to the action of the emetics when a considerable quantity of this poison has been swallowed, perhaps the best means of obviating the evil consequences is the exhibition of an alkaline solution, or a strong solution of soap, if the stomach-pump, which is preferable in the first instance to all other means, cannot be procured. Diffusible stimuli ought to be administered, and cold effusion frequently had recourse to; blood-letting also or blistering, if the head symptoms run high, are advisable. Emollient drinks such as lint-seed tea, thin gum water, sweet milk, &c. are also useful in diminishing irritation.

Belladonna is used as an anodyne, both internally and externally; it has been lately much used in some parts of the continent for the cure of hooping-cough. The cough and other symptoms are said to yield rapidly to its use, but the constitutional excitement caused by the remedy must be continued for some time before a permanent cure can be expected. Amongst the number of its advocates in this disease are Wetzler, Meylin, Hufeland. The greatest caution is requisite in using so violent a remedy where the patients are generally young; the dose is from a quarter to half a grain of the powdered leaves; very gradually increased. Dr M. De Bamberg remarks, that it is principally useful in the primary stage, when there is more or less irritation of the respiratory organs. From the circumstance of Belladonna simulating in its effects some of the symptoms of scarlatina, Dr Hahnemann (author of the homoeopathic system), has introduced it as a preventive when that disease is epidemic; he supposes it to act in the same manner as the vaccine matter does, in preventing the contagion of small-pox, or in modifying the disease when communicated. Many other German physicians corroborate the opinion of Dr Hahnemann. In Toxicological Systems, this plant is referred to the narcotico-acrid section, though the irritating effects are much less obvious than the narcotic; in therapeutic arrangements it is classed under the narcotic.

WOODY NIGHTSHADE OR BITTER-SWEET

Solanum dulcamara

Class and Order, Pentandria Monogynia. Nat. Ord. Solaneæ.

Gen. Char. *Calix* of from five to ten segments; *Corolla* rotate; *Anthers* opening, with two pores at the upper extremity; *Berry* roundish, of two or more cavities.

Root perennial, somewhat creeping; stalk woody, climbing to the height of six feet or more, thinly beset with small-pointed tubercles; leaves on foot-stalks, of an oval pointed shape, extending slightly down the stalks, the lower ones entire, the upper ones lobed or halbert-shaped; flowers on branched cymes; the proper peduncles of the flowers, bulbous at their base, or growing out of a kind of socket; corolla monopetalous, wheel-shaped, the segments turning back; at the bottom of each segment are two roundish green spots, Fig. 3.

The woody nightshade, or, as most commonly called, Dulcamara, was formerly held in considerable repute for medicinal purposes, but at this time has fallen into almost total disuse, though its name is still retained in the modern pharmacopœias. From its berries bearing some resemblance to those of currants, they are often eaten by children, but if speedily removed from the stomach, there is little cause for apprehension.

The natural family of Solaneæ is numerous, and the known species of the present genus amount to perhaps upwards of seventy, yet the whole must be viewed with suspicion, as, though a few species among them afford valuable articles of food, they are all more or less possessed of active poisonous properties, and they are only to be used as food after undergoing some culinary process, by which their noxious qualities are destroyed.

Solanum dulcamara and *nigrum* are held as troublesome weeds, whilst in some other countries the most poisonous of these (*S. nigrum*) is in common use for culinary purposes. The *Solanum tuberosum*, which produces the Potatoe root, is in its wild and uncultivated state not fit for human food; and it is only after a long progress of cultivation that it deleterious qualities are ameliorated. In a raw state it cannot be used as food, but when submitted to the action of heat, it forms a large portion of the food of the peasantry. This useful root abounds in fecula, which is, under peculiar circumstances, entirely converted into a hard gumlike substance; I have a specimen now before me in this state, which has the whole of its interior substance completely changed, whilst the rind retains its usual appearance.

The same difference of opinion exists with regard to the poisonous effect of this as of the *S. nigrum*. Dunal denies it all activity as a poison; but several authors relate cases in which some deleterious effects have been observed. Dr Duncan mentions the following case:—

"A young man affected with a cutaneous complaint had taken the decoction of a handful of the fresh twigs daily for fourteen days without any effect. On the fifteenth, having also taken an ounce of the extract in solution, he was seized with cramps in the calves of his legs, slept during the whole night, but on awaking next morning found his head vacant, vertiginous, *muscæ volitantes*; pupils greatly dilated; cramp of the legs and arms; inability to speak, with stiff swelled tongue; pulse slow and intermitting; cold sweat, and trembling of the limbs. These symptoms soon went off after the administration of a solution of subcarbonate of potass."

This and another case, where a young man became narcotized, and either slept or felt great inclination to do so, for ten hours after merely carrying a bunch of the fresh plant in his hat, (cacuphe) would seem at least to prove that in some constitutions, or under peculiar circumstances, it is not by any means inert. In medicine it is used in scrofula, gout, and chronic rheumatism, in syphilis after the use of mercury, and in cutaneous diseases. It acts as a sudorific and diuretic. The taste is indicated by the specific name; it is first bitter and then sweet.

GARDEN NIGHTSHADE

Solanum nigrum

Class and Order, Natural Order, and Generic Character, see *S. Dulcamara.*

Root annual, branched; stalk one to two feet high, much branched, somewhat angular, from the leaves being decurrent, roughish, a little swollen at the joints; branches alternate; leaves on long foot-stalks, alternate, extending down the stalks, of an oval-pointed form, angularly indented, furnished with a short soft pubescence; flowers growing in a kind of *umbel*; foot-stalks of the flowers spreading, arising from the middle of the stems, between the joints; calix of five ovate segments, which are persistent, and when the fruit is ripe, become black with the berries; corolla wheel-shaped, white, the segments oval and pointed; stamens, five very short hairy filaments; anthers oblong, yellow, somewhat united; pistil, germen roundish and green; style tapering, green, the lower part villous; stigma roundish; seed-vessel a round berry, at first green, when ripe becoming of a deep shining black, with two cavities; seeds several, kidney-shaped, and yellowish.

The *Solanum nigrum*, abounds in neglected gardens, and amongst rubbish, blooming from May to September, and producing its ripe berries about a month after flowering.

The properties of the *Solanum nigrum* have been the cause of much difference of opinion among toxicologists; some asserting it to to be a deadly poison, and others holding it nearly harmless. M. Bourgogne says it is extremely poisonous to sheep, and causes death by its

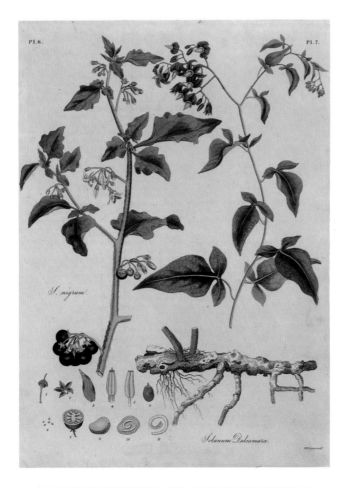

WOODY NIGHTSHADE AND GARDEN NIGHTSHADE

acrid, as well as narcotic effects. In direct opposition to this, we have the experiments of M. Dunal, who not only gave the ripe berries to animals, but ate them himself without observing any bad effects, or suffering any inconvenience. The leaves are used in great quantity as food in the isles of France and Bourbon, and in the Antilles, and are prepared like spinage.

Several cases of poisoning, attributed to the berries of this plant, are mentioned; but, as the *Atropa belladonna* has the same vulgar name as the Solanum, it is more than probable, that the injurious effects ought to be referred to the former plant. Till, however, there is less discrepancy of opinion on the subject, it will be at least safest to regard it with suspicion.

Solanine was discovered in 1821 by M. Desfosses in the *S. nigrum* and *dulcamara*; by Morin it was found in *S. mammosum*; by Pelletier and Payen in the berries of the *Verbascifolium*, an American plant; it is not used in medicine. Orfila says, that it is more emetic in its properties than opium, and not so soothing.

Berzelius mentions, with some expression of doubt, its existence in the *S. tuberosum* as discovered by Baup.

MEZEREON OR SPURGE LAUREL

Daphne mezereum

Class and Order, Octandria Monogynia. Nat. Ord. Thymeleæ.
Gen. Char. *Perianth* single, inferior, like a corolla, quadripartite. *Berry* with one seed.

THE Mezereon forms a low bushy shrub, and is to be found in most gardens, where it is cultivated for its early blossoming and the delightful fragrance of its flowers: it has been admitted into the British Flora, though it can scarcely be considered a native; the few situations in which it has been found growing apparently wild, would induce a belief that it had by some means escaped from gardens. I feel confirmed in this opinion from having found it in the spring of 1832, growing on a rock at a considerable elevation: on climbing to the spot I found a considerable number of the seeds and half-digested berries, also some young seedlings of perhaps a year old, and subsequently noticed the berries to be eaten by blackbirds and thrushes,

which may account for the seeds being found in the above named situation, which was much resorted to by various species of thrush.

D. laureola is equally acrid with *D. mezereum*, and the berries are stated by De Candolle to be poisonous to all animals excepting birds; the berries of the Mezereon are extremely acrid, and have frequently proved highly injurious, though eaten in but very small quantities.

The flowers grow in thick clusters and near the extremities of the branches, appearing before the expansion of the leaves, and are succeeded by their bright scarlet fruit, which arrives at maturity in the summer months.

The natural family of the Thymeleæ, to which the *Mezereon* belongs, are remarkable for the extreme acridity of their bark and roots. For this reason, the various species are not much used in medicine; the *D. Mezereum* is the only one mentioned in our pharmacopœias, and its use is much circumscribed, the sequela of syphilis and scrofula being the only cases in which it is employed. Its action is sudorific and alternative, but it is seldom given alone; in combination with Sarsaparilla, Sassafras, Guaiac and Liquorice, it

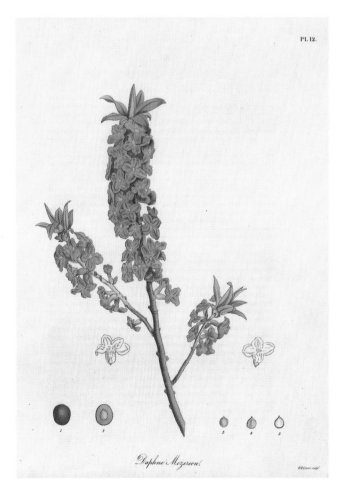

Pl. 12.

Daphne Mezereon

SPURGE LAUREL OR MEZEREON

forms the *Decoctum Sarsaparilla Compositum,* a preparation resembling the celebrated Lisbon Diet Drink, and very useful in the sequela of syphilis, either after, or along with, a mercurial course; whether this preparation owes much of its efficacy to the Mezereon is to be doubted.

In France the *Daphne gnidium* or *Garou,* is used instead of the Mezereon. The external application of this species as an epispastic, is recommended by some in cases where cantharides is inadmissible, and a formula for a preparation of an ointment, (*Pommade du Garou*) is given; 4 parts of the root bruised and moistened, are to be boiled in a mixture of 10 parts of hog's lard, with 2 of wax, till all the moisture be dissipated. Instead of this ointment, the French apothecaries sell another under the same name, of which cantharides is the active ingredient, but prepared in such a manner as seldom to give rise to any unpleasant symptoms.

EUROPEAN OLIVE

Olea europea

Class and Order, DIANDRIA **M**ONOGYNIA. **N**AT. **O**RD. **O**LEACEÆ.
Gen. Char. *Corolla* and *Calix* four cleft: *Drupe* superior, one-seeded: *Embryo* inverse, and furnished with a perisperm. *Schreb.*

———

THE Olive is a native of the warmer parts of Europe, where it is extensively cultivated for its fruit; it forms a tree from twenty to thirty feet high; the leaves are thick and lance-shaped, and as well as the flowers much resemble those of the common Privet, but the flowers grow in denser but smaller racemes; the fruit is a berry of the size of a large hazel nut, at first green, and when ripe of a purplish colour; in the unripe state they are pickled in salt and water, and are used at our tables, rather to excite thirst, than from any agreeable or pleasant taste. Professor Lindley remarks, "that this order offers almost the only instance of oil being contained in the pericarp, from which olive oil is entirely expressed."

Though sufficiently hardy to bear our winters in sheltered situations, the olive rarely produces fruit in this country; it has been cultivated in England since the year 1648. One species, the *O. fragrans,* is used in China for the purpose of giving a flavour to some particular kinds of tea.

The best olive oil is prepared by the simple expression of the fruit, which has remained in heaps for thirteen or fourteen days, or which has begun to show the signs of fermentation. Inferior oils are obtained by allowing the fermentation to proceed till the mucilage be destroyed, or by throwing the fruit into boiling water, before submitting it to pressure.

When taken internally, olive oil acts as a laxative; it is, however, seldom used; as an external application it is occasionally employed. In poisoning with acrid substances, it is extremely useful as an internal remedy; it is also given as an injection in cases of ileus, and in painful ulceration of the rectum.

Dr Bidot, Physician to the military hospital at Loning, has lately proposed the dried leaves of the olive as a substitute for quinine in intermittent fever, but trials, which have been made of its efficacy in La Charité, though they proved that it was not without effect, yet in their results fell short of what had been stated by Dr Bidot.

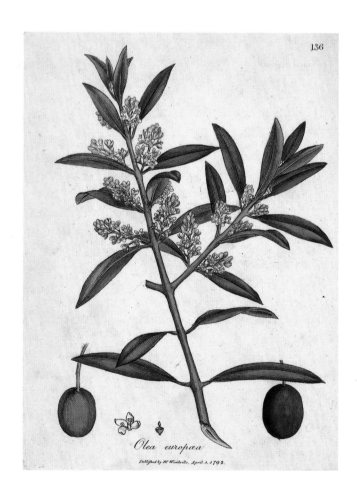

EUROPEAN OLIVE

COMMON FLAX

Linum usitatissimum

Class and Order, Pentandria Pentagynia. Nat. Ord. Lineæ.
Gen. Char. *Calix* of five persistent leaves; *Petals* five; *Capsule* globose, mucronate, with ten valves, and ten cells; *Seeds* ovate, compressed.

Root annual, fibrous; stalks upright, a foot or two high or more, round, smooth, leafy, branching only at the top; leaves lanceolate, sessile, at the lower part of the stem growing thickly together, without any order, on the upper part of the stem more distant and alternate; flowers large, of a delicate purplish blue colour; petals five, wedge-shaped, deciduous, streaked with veins of a deeper colour, the tips notched as if eaten by insects, the claws white.

Flax, though enumerated among our indigenous plants, is but a doubtful native, yet, from the length of time it has been cultivated, its seeds have become disseminated, and it is generally esteemed an aborigine. It is a hardy annual of considerable beauty, and is cultivated in most countries of Europe for the fibres afforded by its stems, known by the common appellation of flax or lint; as also for its seeds. Their uses in domestic economy and the arts are numerous.

In addition to its extensive use in the arts, the *Linum usitatissimum* is employed in medicine in several forms. The infusion of the seed is one of our most useful mucilaginous drinks, and is employed in inflammatory diseases, in diarrhœa, and in all irritations of the alimentary canal; from the diuretic property which the infusion possesses, it is also used in diseases of the bladder and in strangury arising from any accidental circumstances; in chronic diarrhœa, much relief is often afforded by an injection, composed of the infusion combined with laudanum. In surgical practice, the farinaceous part of the seeds, under the name of lintseed meal, is very generally used for making poultices, and in combination with the decoction of poppies, as a sedative poultice to irritable or cancerous sores. The oil is also employed as an external application in burns, and when formed into a liniment with lime-water forms the well known Carron Oil.

Lintseed oil is seldom used internally, as there are so many much less nauseous fixed oils in common use. As an injection in ileus, and spasmodic contractions of the intestines, it is occasionally used. In poisoning with acrid substances, and especially with the alkalies, this, or any other bland fixed oil, is very useful.

To procure the oil, the seeds are first roasted to deprive them of as much mucilage as possible; they are then moistened with hot water and subjected to pressure; the oil thus obtained is of a greenish yellow colour, and usually of a rancid disagreeable taste. The cake which remains after the expression of the oil, is called Oil-Cake, and is used for fattening cattle. Lintseed oil when exposed to the air, absorbs oxygen, and becomes dry and almost resinous in appearance; from this property it is called a drying oil. The combination between the oxygen and the oil is occasionally so rapid, as to cause a rise of temperature sufficient to set fire to dry vegetable substances; hence have arisen several destructive fires in cotton manufactories and in flax and cordage stores. With litharge, this oil enters into chemical union, and acquires the property of drying in a remarkable degree; in this state it is used by painters.

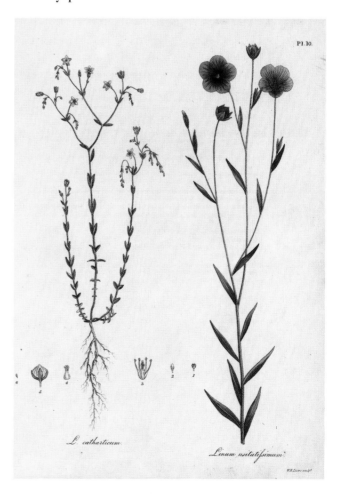

COMMON FLAX AND PURGING FLAX

Printers also use it for making printing ink; they prepare it by boiling, inflaming and allowing it to burn till it has acquired the proper consistence.

PURGING FLAX

Linum catharticum

Class and Order, Natural Order, and Generic Character, see *L. usitatissimum.*

ROOT annual and fibrous; stalks from three inches to a foot or more high, upright, smooth, round, and branched at the top; leaves opposite, nearly upright, smooth, perfectly entire, on the upper parts of the branches alternate and lanceolate; flowers white, before expanding drooping; petals white, spreading, pointed, slightly united at the base, having three ribs and yellow claws.

This small but elegant species of flax is dispersed over Great Britain. It abounds on chalky and hilly districts, also amongst sand on the sea shore; in the last situation, we have found it attaining a large size than we have ever seen it under any circumstances,—having gathered it on the shores of the Firth of Forth nearly two feet high. It is sometimes found growing in meadows; flowers from June to August, and ripens its seed about a month or five weeks after blooming; and it continues a long time in flower, it often happens that unopen buds, fully expanded blossoms, and ripe capsules, are at the same time met with on the same plant.

Though retained in our Pharmacopœias, the *Linum catharticum* is rarely used in regular practice; it is possessed, however, of strongly marked purgative properties, and forms an exception to the character for blandness, for which the natural family of the *Lineæ* is distinguished. Another species, the *L. selaginoides,* is said to be bitter and aperient. The usual mode in which the *L. catharticum* is exhibited, is by infusing a handful of the fresh herb in whey, and drinking the infusion while warm. The country people consider this as useful as many of our more costly medicines.

DANDELION

Leontodon taraxacum

Class and Order, SYNGENESIA ÆQUALIS. NAT. ORD. COMPOSITÆ.
Gen. Char. *Involucre* imbricated with scales, the outermost frequently reflexed; *Receptacle* naked; *Pappus* stipitate, simple.

ROOT perennial, milky. penetrating to a considerable depth; leaves more or less deeply jagged or toothed, each tooth pointed and sharply indented; stalks naked, hollow, each supporting one flower; the common or general calix smooth; the lowermost leaves or *squamæ* turning back; flower large and shewy; seed a little crooked, flattish and somewhat four-cornered, grooved, at the top prickly; down or pappus standing on a footstalk, simple; receptacle naked, full of holes.

A most abundant species, common to fields, hedge banks, and uncultivated places, flowering in May and continuing the whole summer. Its parts of fructification being conspicuous, it offers to the young botanist a good example of the structure of compound flowers.

In Europe the *Leontodon taraxacum* has been in vogue as a tonic and alternative; in France, it is much used in chronic diseases of the skin and in visceral obstructions; the dose given is from two or three ounces of the expressed juice.

Richard remarks that it is one of those remedies which insensibly alters the state of the system. I have seen it used with good effect (in combination with the Dulcamara) instead of sarsaparilla.

The young leaves are eaten as salad, but when mature, their bitterness is too intense to allow of their being used in this way.

The root, flower-stems, and leaves abound with a milky juice, which has the property of causing a permanent dark-coloured stain on the skin and on linen. John has found that caoutchouc, resin, gum, bitter extractive, sugar, a free acid, and salts of lime and potass are contained in the fresh juice. Inuline has been procured from the fresh root by Waltt in the proportion of half an ounce from a pound.

Pl. 9.

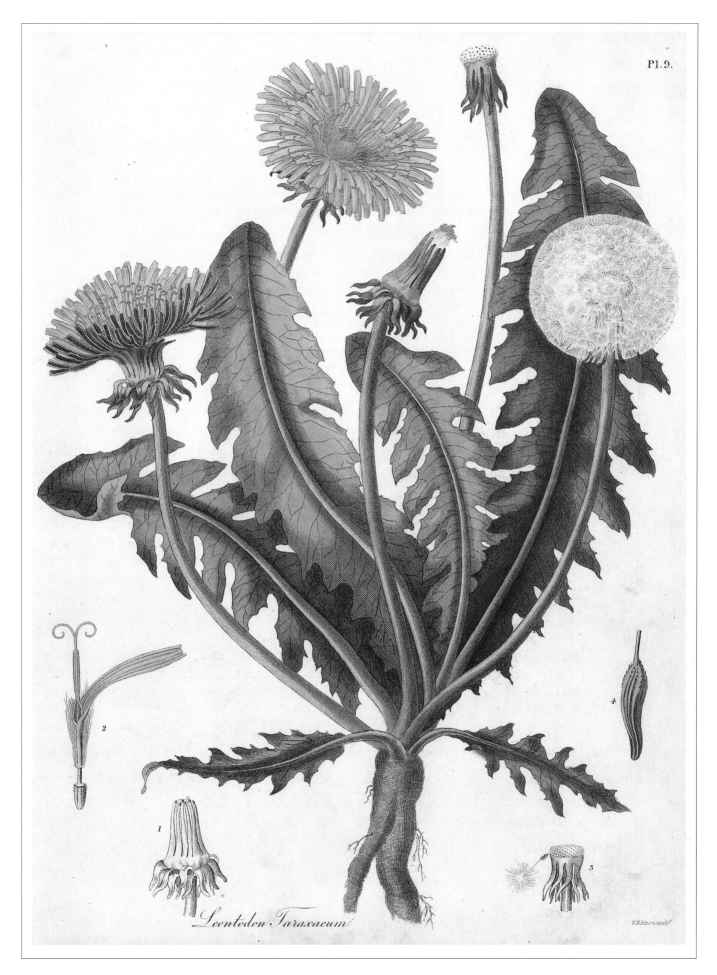

Leontodon Taraxacum

DANDELION

BLACK PEPPER

Piper nigrum

Class and Order, Diandria Trigynia. Nat. Ord. Piper-
aceæ.
Gen. Char. *Calix* and *Corolla* wanting; *Berry* one-seeded;
Spadix simple.

This well known species is a native of the East Indies, and the islands of Sumatra, Java, Borneo, and the Phillipines; it is a climbing plant, growing to the length of eight or ten feet, its root is perennial, stems round, smooth and jointed, becoming tumid at the joints, woody, straggling and branching; leaves broadly ovate, pointed, entire, smooth, having seven nerves, of a full green colour; flowers in a lax spike, placed on a longish peduncle, which grows opposite the leaves, and alternates with them.

Black pepper is cultivated in the stoves of this country, but we can rarely perfect its fruit, which when ripe is of a deep scarlet colour, and has a very elegant appearance, and is prepared for use by rubbing off the skin when perfectly dry; the berries then become black and shrivelled. White pepper is prepared by macerating the black pepper in water until the outer skin separates; it is afterwards dried, and in the operation loses some of its pungency. This genus contains a great number of species, the whole of which are possessed of the same properties in a greater or lesser degree.

Black pepper is extensively used as a condiment, and from its stimulating power is useful in aiding digestion in phlegmatic habits. When taken habitually and in quantity, it is apt to cause visceral derangement. The taste of this spice is warm and fiery; its odour is aromatic. It exerts a powerful action on the animal economy, causing increased action of the heart and arteries, and when taken in large quantity, producing all the symptoms of irritant poisoning. Dr Christison quotes from Rust's Journal, the case of a man who, from taking between an ounce and a half and two ounces in brandy, was attacked with convulsions, burning heat of the throat and stomach, great thirst, and vomiting of everything he swallowed. His case was treated as one of simple gastritis, and he recovered. The fiery, acrid taste depends on a fixed oil, and the stimulating property is also referred to it, but since the discovery of Piperine, much difference of opinion has existed on this subject. The power which pepper possesses of reddening and inflaming the skin, resides in the fixed oil.

Pepper has long been a popular remedy in agues and fevers of all descriptions, and much mischief occasionally arises from its injudicious use in this way. Besides Piperine and fixed oil, pepper contains a balsamic volatile oil; a gummy colouring substance; extractive analogous to that of leguminous plants; bassorine; malic and uric acids; lignine, and various earthy salts.

LONG PEPPER

Piper longum

Class, Order, Nat. Ord. and Generic Character, see *P.*
nigrum.

This species, like the preceding one, is a native of the East Indies, and the islands in the Indian Archipelago; it is easily distinguished from *P. nigrum*, by its cordate leaves and dense pikes; its berries are very small, and the whole plant possesses the same properties as the *nigrum*. Though sometimes used in medicine, it is more generally applied to culinary purposes as a condiment.

The *Piper longum* differs but little in its medicinal virtues from the *nigrum*; it is less aromatic, and more acrid. The analysis by Dulong D'Astafort is nearly the same as that given under the head of *Piper nigrum*; in addition to the substances there mentioned, it is said by him to contain fecula and vegetable mucilage. Berzelius regards what is called fixed oil in this, and the preceding plant, as resin.

CUBEBS OR JAVA PEPPER

Piper cubeba

Class and Order, Nat. Ord. and Generic Character, see
P. nigrum.

The Isle of Java, and other parts of the East Indies, produce the official Cubebs, which grows to a considerable size; the leaves grow singly, and are placed opposite the spikes of flowers, which are very small, closely crowded in spikes, and are succeeded by berries of a dull scarlet, placed on short foot-stalks; the fruit is globular, smooth, fleshy, becoming brown in drying.

Though long used by the native practitioners of India for the cure of gonorrhœa, Cubebs was not employed in Europe till after the year 1818; when a paper, containing an account of the benefit derived from the remedy by the Hindoos, verified by the experience of the author, and other British medical men resident in Java, was published by Mr Crawfurd. Cubebs, like the other peppers, is a powerful excitant, but its stimulating effects rapidly disappear, and its specific power of exciting the kidneys and urinary passages becomes manifest. In cases of gonorrhœa, in which constitutional excitement is considerable, and accompanied by inflammatory fever, Cubebs ought not to be used; it is when the consitutional disturbance has abated, or in forms of the disease in which there has not been any febrile excitement, that benefit is to be expected from its exhibition. The use of this remedy ought to be continued for some time after the discharge has ceased, as the disease is otherwise apt to return.

SAFFRON CROCUS

Crocus sativus

Class and Order, TRIANDRIA MONOGYNIA. NAT. ORD. IRIDEÆ.
Gen. Char. *Perianth* coloured; *tube* very long; *limb* cut into six equal segments. *Stigma* three-lobed, plaited.

ROOT bulbous, thickly covered with a loose reticulated skin; leaves long, deep green, with a whitish line passing up the centre of each; flowers growing from a thin transparent sheath; tube, filaments, and pistil long, often attaining six or eight inches in length; the leaves appear early in September, and the flowers about the end of or beginning of October. It increases rapidly by its roots, is a beautiful and very delicate flower, well meriting a place in every garden.

The stigmas of this species produce the saffron of the shops, and the plants are extensively cultivated for this drug, in various parts of England, but it may be doubted if it is truly a native. The saffron is collected and kept closely packed, and either formed into what is termed cakes, or hay saffron; the latter is generally the most pure, any adulteration being more easily detected in this state than when compressed into cakes. When of good quality it has a strong fragrant smell, inclining to aromatic, a warm taste, and readily imparts a beautiful golden yellow colour to boiling water.

Saffron possesses considerable power as an excitant; in small doses it is tonic and stimulating; in larger, antispasmodic, and sedative; in an overdose it produces all the symptoms of intoxication. In France, it it chiefly used as an emmenagogue; in this country, it is seldom used in an uncombined form in medicine. When taken habitually, it colours the perspiration, saliva, and urine yellow, and imparts to them its peculiar odour.

Saffron owes it medicinal and odoriferous qualities to an essential oil; its colouring power depends on a principle, discovered by Bouillon Lagrange and Vogel, and named by them Polychroite. It is procured by digesting saffron in water, and evaporating the solution to the consistence of extract, by exhausting the extract with alcohol, and evaporating to dryness; the substance which remains is Polychroite, combined with volatile oil.

COMMON GINGER

Zingiber officinale

Class and Order, MONANDRIA MONOGYNIA. NAT. ORD. SCITAMINEÆ.
Gen. Char. *Corolla* with the interior border umbilicate; *Anther* double, crowned with a single horn-shaped curved beak; *Capsule* three-celled, three-valved; *Seeds* many, arilled; *Embryo* simple, and furnished with both *Perisperm* and *Vitellus*, *Fl. Ind.*

ROOT biennial or perennial, forming hard, knotty, compressed tubers, from which arise a number of round, erect stalks from two to four feet high, which are annual, and are enveloped in smooth membranous sheaths; leaves alternate, of a deep bright green colour, smooth, long and terminating in long narrow points: flower-stalks from six inches to a foot long, enveloped in a few obtuse sheaths, which on the upper part elongate into leaves: Flowers in a dense spike; exterior segments of a pale yellow colour; lip purple with yellow spots.

In the late Mr Roscoe's superb publication of the plants of this natural order, are figured nine species of this curious genus, and in the Flora Indica eleven are enumerated, many of which are now cultivated in this kingdom. They are all natives of the warmer parts of Asia and America.

In the East and West Indies, the common ginger is grown extensively for its roots, which are exported, either dry, (the ginger of commerce) or in a green state preserved in sugar.

Ginger affords an excellent example of underground stems, *Rhizoma* of modern botanists, being what are generally denominated roots; but the true roots are the fibres only which grow from these parts, in a similar manner with those of the most familiar genus, Iris. Most of the plants constituting this natural family are aromatic, and all the species are highly interesting, either from the singularity of structure, or elegance of their flowers, also from affording a considerable number of useful drugs.

The two kinds of Ginger, which are sold under the names of black, and white, are the produce of the same plants, and of the same gathering. The black is prepared by being immersed in boiling water, and dried; the white, by being deprived of its skin, and dried in the sun. As the best roots are selected for the latter, the white ginger is found to be stronger than the black, and sells at a higher price. In medicine, the white is commonly used; for domestic and culinary purposes, the black is more frequently employed. Ginger is a stimulant tonic, and is useful in aiding digestion in phlegmatic habits; in dyspepsia, arising from the torpid action of the stomach and bowels, and in flatulent colic, it is also useful. Some authors recommend its employment in gout. The effect on the circulation is not so powerful, as the pungent taste and tonic properties would lead us to suppose; Ginger differs from cayenne, and some other spices, in causing a sensation of heat in the stomach, which they, though they as powerfully affect the mouth and throat, do not occasion. Ginger is exhibited in the form of tincture, powder, or lozenge. An empirical preparation under the name of "Oxley's essence of ginger," has acquired considerable celebrity, and is, I believe, a very good form of administering this drug.

Richard says, "the English prepare from the Ginger a very exciting beverage, which they call Ginger-Beer."

LESSER CARDAMOM

Alpinia cardamomum

Class and Order, MONADRIA MONOGYNIA. NAT. ORD. SCITAMINEÆ.
Gen. Char. *Corolla* with the interior border unilabiate; *Anther* double, naked; *Capsule* berried, three-celled; *Seeds* few or many, arilled; *Embryo* simple, and furnished with both *Perisperm* and *Vitellus. Schreber.*

FROM the synonyms it will be observed that the structure of this flower was not clearly understood, or presented so anomalous a structure as to render its proper station dubious; but it now appears judiciously placed, in the Flora Indica of the late Dr Roxburgh, in the genus *Alpinia*.

Root perennial, creeping, tuberous with fleshy fibres; stems perennial, erect, smooth, jointed, enveloped in the spongy sheaths of the leaves, from six to nine feet high; leaves bifarious, subsessile on their sheaths, lanceolate, fine pointed, somewhat villous above, resinous underneath, entire; length from one to two feet; sheath slightly villous, with a round stipulary process rising above the mouth; scapes several, from the base of the stems, resting on the ground, flexuose, jointed, ramous, from one to two feet long. Flowers alternate, inner lip or nectary obovate and much longer than the divisions of the exterior border; margins somewhat curled, with the apex slightly three-lobed,

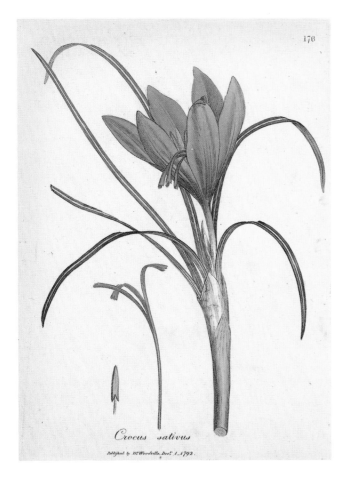

Crocus sativus

Published by J. Woodville, Dec.r 1, 1792.

SAFFRON CROCUS

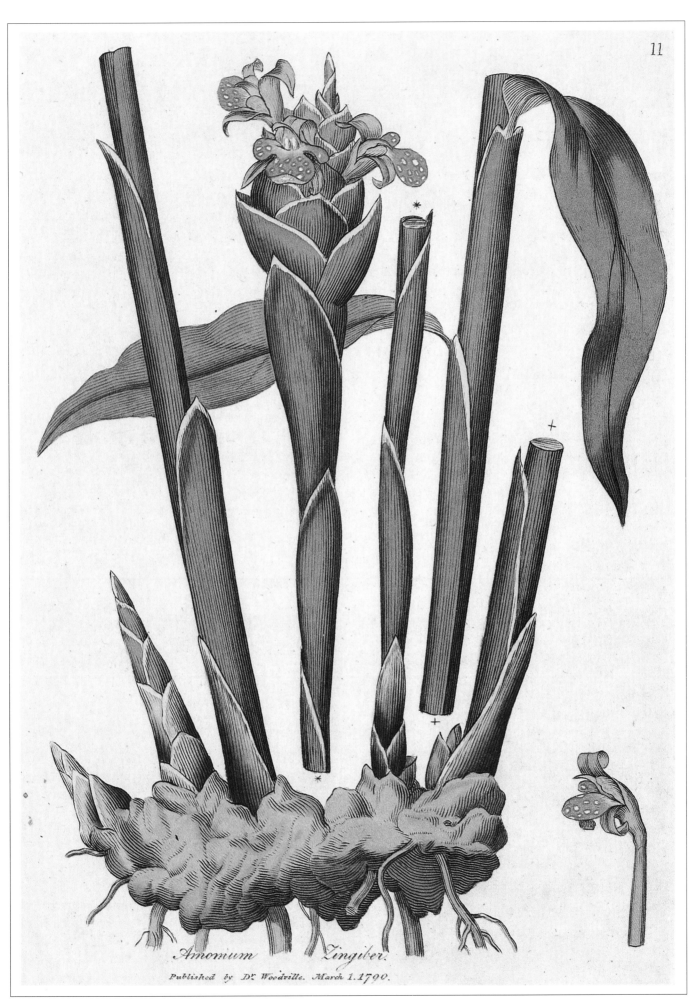

Amomum Zingiber.

Published by Dᵣ Woodville. March 1. 1790.

COMMON GINGER

marked chiefly in the centre with violet stripes, at each side of its insertion, and close by the base of the filament is a small acute hornlet, as in most of the plants in this genus, and in several other genera of our other Indian Scitamineæ.—*Flora Indica.*

This interesting plant belongs to a genus containing some of the most splendid productions of the vegetable kindgom, as the *A. nutans, auriculata,* &c. Its seeds, which are the only officinal part of the plant, are highly aromatic, and are known in the shops by the name of Cardamoms; when good and fresh they are of a dark but bright brown colour, and possess an agreeable warm aromatic flavour, which they retain more completely when imported in the capsule, and speedily lose it when exposed to the air.

Dr Roxburgh enumerates twelve species of this genus, all natives of India. "The *cardamomum* shrub is found in great abundance among the western mountains of Mynaad, and is called by the natives of Malabar *Ailum chedy* (the ailum shrub.) The seeds of the *Amomum cardamomum* are of an agreeable aromatic taste, and are used by the Malays as a substitute for the Cardamom of Malabar."

The seeds of the Cardamom are used in medicine chiefly in combination with other aromatic tonics; they are useful in colic arising from flatulence, and in the dyspepsia of weak habits; they form agreeable additions to some other tonics, and cover the taste of some nauseous drugs. The compound tincture of Cardamom was recommended in the first stage of cholera, and was occasionally useful in arresting the nausea, and in relieving the pain of the stomach and the bowels. In the common cholera of this country, the compound tincture of Cardamom or of Cinnamon, when combined with a few drops of laudanum, often completely cuts short the symptoms.

HEDGE HYSSOP

Gratiola officinalis

Class and Order, Diandria Monogynia. Nat. Ord. Scrophularæ.
Gen. Char. *Corolla* one-petalled, irregular; *Sterile filaments* two, affixed to the lower lip of the corolla; *Anthers* double, and connected; *Capsule* superior, two-celled, two-valved; *Seeds* numerous. *Schreb.*

A NATIVE of the south of Europe, affecting wet situations and of easy culture. In the *Flora Indica*, Dr Roxburgh describes eighteen species as natives of India, and one is found in Virginia, all of which, like the European species, delight in moist situations.

Root perennial, whitish, fibrous; stem simple, round, erect, about a foot high; leaves sessile, opposite, lanceolate, serrated from about the centre to the points; flowers growing from the base of the leaves, of a pale purple colour, streaked with darker veins; tube yellowish; filaments four, of which only two are furnished with anthers; capsule of two cells; seeds numerous. All the species are possessed of a bitter nauseous taste; and Rumphius remarks, "that the leaves of *G. amara* are exceedingly bitter, and might, no doubt, answer valuable purposes in medicine."

The *Gratiola officinalis* is occasionally used by the poorer classes as a cathartic; when taken in a small quantity, it acts as a drastic purgative, frequently causing nausea; when taken in an over-dose, all the symptoms of acrid poisoning are produced.

Orfila gives an account of several cases, in which nymphomania was caused by injections prepared from this plant.

Gleditsch has observed that horses which are fed on hay containing much of the Gratiola soon became lean.

OFFICINAL OR WILD VALERIAN

Valeriana officinalis

Class and Order, Triandria Monogynia. Nat. Ord. Valerianeæ.
Gen. Char. *Calix* a thickened margin to the top of the germen, at length unfolding into a feathery pappus; *Corolla* monopetalous, five cleft, gibbous or spurred at the base; *Fruit* one-seeded, crowned with the feathery *Pappus. Hooker.*

THE Valerian is an indigenous plant of common occurrence, being usually found in low moist situations, but sometimes affecting more elevated and drier places; in the latter situations, the root (which is the officinal part of the plant,) is possessed of much more powerful properties than when growing in wet spots. There is also much difference in the appearance of the plant in these various places of growth, the leaves being broader, and the plants more robust, when growing in watery than on dry places.

For medicinal purposes the roots should not be taken up during their greenest state, as their peculiar odour is much more powerful towards the close of autumn and during winter, than at other periods.

When cultivated in gardens, the Valerian is liable to be injured by cats, which are so partial to the smell that it is used occasionally as a bait to decoy them into traps,.

Twenty species are enumerated in Loudon's *Hortus Britannicus*, and two others in the *Flora Indica*.

The action of Valerian on the system is first stimulant, then antispasmodic and sedative. In nervous diseases, and in fever, it is frequently administered, and is one of the most useful and powerful antispasmodics which the vegetable kingdom affords; the taste of the root, which is the only part used in medicine, is bitter, and slightly acrid; its smell strong and disagreeable. Its virtues depend on a volatile oil, which possesses its odour in a concentrated degree; this oil is most abundant, and the root consequently most active, when the plant has grown in a dry elevated situation. Though the smell of Valerian be considered disagreeable by Europeans, some species are used in the east for the purpose of perfuming baths. The *V. jatamensi* is supposed to be the true spikenard, and is valued in India both for its odour and medicinal properties. Cats are very fond of the smell of Valerian, and are thrown into a sort of intoxication by it; the male is more affected by it than the female. In Sicily, the young leaves of the red valerian are used as salad, and an allied genus, the Valerianella, (lamb's lettuce,) furnishes several plants, the leaves of which are considered, by some, equal to those of the *Lactuca sativa*, (garden lettuce.)

COMMON ROSEMARY

Rosmarinus officinalis

Class and Order, Diandria Monogynia. Nat. Ord. Labiatæ.
Gen. Char. *Corolla* unequal, with the upper lip two-pointed; *Filaments* long, curved; *Stigma* toothed.

THIS shrub is a native of the south of Europe, but is quite hardy, and thrives well in cooler climates; it grows to the height of from three to six feet; the branches are straggling and covered with a loose greyish bark; leaves growing in whorls, long, narrow, rigid, obtuse; of a dark green on the upper side, beneath silvery grey; flowers growing from the axils of the leaves; of a pale blue colour with white blotches.

Rosemary was introduced into England in the year 1598; it grows wild in the southern provinces of France, but more abundantly in Spain, Italy, and the Levant.

The smell of the Rosemary is strong and fragrant, and bears a slight resemblance to that of lavender, but is not nearly so pleasant. The taste is pungent, bitter, and aromatic. It is often used in medicine, but possesses powerfully stimulating properties.

The taste, odour, and medicinal qualities, reside in an essential oil, which pervades every part of the plant. It is very acrid, and is seldom given in an uncombined form; it contains a considerable quantity of camphor, which is deposited in a crystallized state, if the oil be allowed to remain at rest for a length of time; it differs from the other volatile oils, in not being easily decomposed by the sulphuric or nitric acids. It is one of the principal ingredients, in the preparation known by the name of "Hungary water," and it also enters into the composition of *Eau de Cologne*.

FLORENTINE IRIS OR SWEET ORRIS

Iris florentina

Class and Order, Triandria Monogynia. Nat. Ord. Ensatæ, Lin, Irideæ, Brown.
Gen. Char. *Perianth* single, petaloid, six-cleft, each alternate segment longer and reflexed; *Stigmas* three, petaloid, covering the stamens.

THIS handsome species, which was cultivated by Gerard in 1596, in a native of Italy, and, like most of the genus, thrives exceedingly in temperate climates, so as frequently to become troublesome in gardens. Root large, tuberous, compressed, fibrous, externally brown, within of a pale yellowish-white colour; flowers large, of a delicate pale-blue tint.

Orris root is chiefly used as a perfume; it enters into the composition of most dentifrices, and into many of the essences prepared for the toilet; its smell resembles that of the *Viola odorata*, and its tincture is sold under the name of Essence of violets.

In doses of from twelve to twenty grains, it is said to be useful in chronic catarrhs, and in asthma. Small pieces of the root, cut of the size and into the form of a pea, are used for the purpose of keeping issues open; besides their mechanical effect, some benefit is supposed to arise from the stimulating property which they possess. A spirituous liquor made by digesting Orris root in proof spirit, to which a little sugar has been added, is sold as *Brandy*.

According to Vogel, the Orris root contains a volatile oil; nearly solid, of a pale yellow colour, and of a fragrant odour; starch; gum; extractive matter; a fixed oil, or rather a resin, bitter and acrid; woody fibre.

RHATTANY

Krameria triandria

Class and Order, Tetrandria Monogynia. Ord. Polygaleæ.
Gen. Char. *Calix* of four or five segments, silky outside; *Petals* four or five, two of which are orbicular, the third constantly of two or three united petals, all unguiculate; *Stamens* three or four, free from the base; *Anthers* bursting by two pores; *Fruit* one-celled, one-seeded, globose, indehiscent, echinated.—*Don.*

Rhattany is a native of Peru, growing in the declivities of sandy mountains, from whence its roots are gathered in large quantities and exported into Europe; from which a deep red colour is obtained, and is principally used in the manufacture of Port wine. So important were its uses considered, that the Spanish and Portuguese merchants have kept its properties so concealed, that in this country the root was unknown till very lately. It forms a low shrub, scarcely exceeding one foot in height.

Rhattany root was first introduced into European practice by Ruiz, one of the authors of the *Flora of Peru*; he recommended it in leucorrhœa, in hæmorrhages, in obstinate diarrhœa; and, in short, in all cases in which astringent tonics were indicated. Subsequent trials have verified M. Ruiz's statements. The Rhattany may be exhibited in the form of decoction, extract, or tincture; the extract which is prepared in America, is, of course, liable to adulteration, and is consequently variable in its strength. This, as well as kino, is used for the adulteration of Port wine,

and from the astringency of its taste, and the deep red colour which it imparts, it is well suited for the purpose. The Peruvians use the Rhattany as a dentifrice, and it is now pretty often employed in a similar manner, in this country.

SCARLET PIMPERNEL OR POOR MAN'S WEATHER-GLASS

Anagallis arvensis

Class and Order, Pentandria Monogynia. Nat. Ord. Primulaceæ.
Gen. Char. *Calix* of five segments; *Corolla* rotate; *Stamens* hairy; *Capsule* bursting transversely.

This beautiful annual is common to most parts of Britain and is well known for the beauty of its blossoms, as well as from the circumstance of its closing its flowers previous to and during damp weather, whence its common English name. It varies in the colour of its flowers, being usually of a deep scarlet, sometimes pure white, or pink, and I am inclined to believe the *A. cærulea* is only a variety of the present species. It was formerly held in esteem for medical purposes, but has fallen into disuse; yet, as some instances are recorded of serious accidents having arisen from its leaves having been inadvertently eaten, it is enumerated as a species rather to be classed with the suspected, than known poisonous plants.

The *Anagallis arvenis* is not used in medicine. Guillemin, in the *Dictionnaire des Drogues*, states that some practitioners have held it up as a specific in madness, but he gives it as his opinion, that not the least reliance is to be placed on these assertions. In this opinion most medical men will, I think coincide.

BROAD-LEAVED WATER PARSNEP

Sium latifolium

Class and Order, Pentandria Digynia. Nat. Ord. Umbelliferæ.
Gen. Char. *Fruit* nearly ovate, compressed, striated; *Involucre* of many leaves; *Petals* cordate, uniform.

Root creeping, perennial; stems from three to six feet high, branched, hollow, smooth, deeply grooved and angular; leaves large, those growing under water often deeply cut, those above

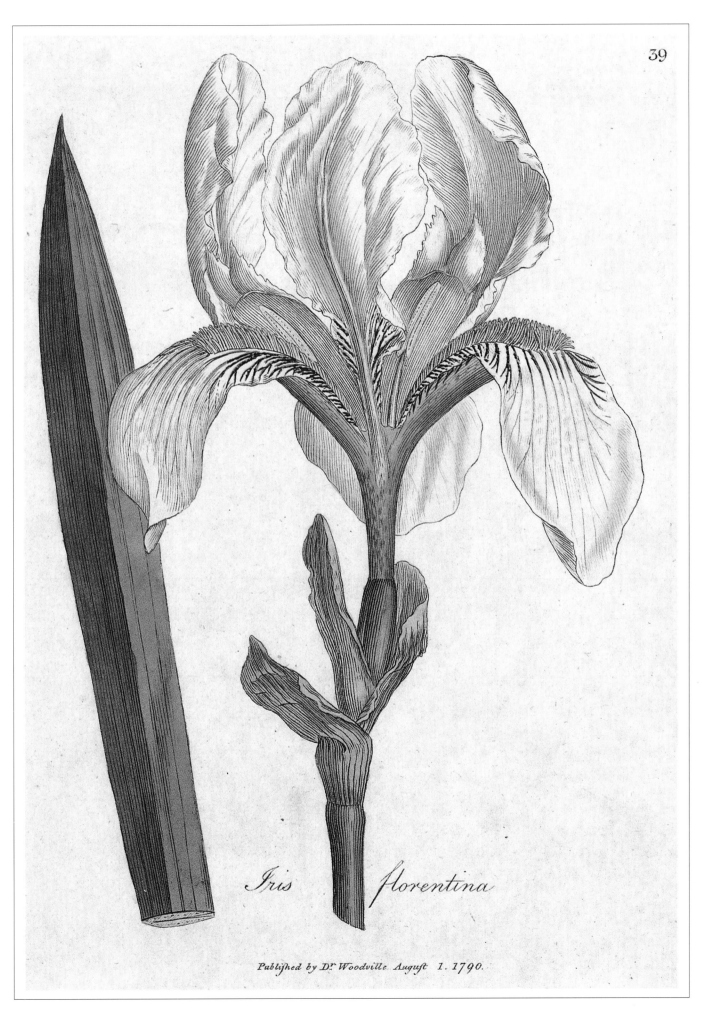

Iris florentina

Published by Dr Woodville August 1. 1790.

FLORENTINE IRIS OR SWEET ORRIS

narrower, shorter, with fewer leaflets and more acute; petioles with a membranous sheath.

A common inhabitant of ditches and marshy places, increasing rapidly by its roots. The leaves which are sometimes consumed by cattle are very injurious, and in some instances, where they have been inadvertently eaten as water-cresses, have proved nearly fatal. It bears a close resemblance to the next species, but is easily known by the broad sheaths to the foot-stalks.

NARROW-LEAVED WATER PARSNEP

Sium angustifolium

Class and Order, Nat. Ord. and Gen. Char. See *S. latifolium.*

ROOT perennial and creeping; stems three or four feet high, erect, branched, hollow, round, and but slightly striated; leaves alternate, pinnate, with a single leaflet at the point, the lower ones the largest. This is a more slender plant than the preceding, and is readily distinguished by its smaller and unequally cut leaves, and by the sheaths of the stalks.

Its properties are considered as identical with those of the *S. latifolium*, but more active: some fatal accidents are recorded from the leaves having been eaten as cresses. Till more certain information is obtained relative to their noxious properties, it will be prudent to avoid the whole of our native species, though it may eventually prove that the injurious qualities attributed to the Siums really belong to some other genus.

Some doubt seems to exist, as to the properties of the plants forming this genus; the two species above described, are said to be poisonous; the *Sium nodiflorum* is given in very large doses as a diuretic, (4 fl. oz. of the juice of the fresh root in milk.) The *S. sisarum* or *Skirret* is stated to be nutritious and wholesome. The *S. ninsi* was supposed to be the plant which produced the celebrated Ginseng of the Chinese, a medicine, which they employ in all diseases, and which the Emperor in 1709, sent an army to obtain. But though the Ginseng is now known to be the produce of the *Panax quinquefolium*, yet we find the *S. ninsi* cultivated in China as an excitant. The *S. sisarum*, according to Berzelius, does not essentially differ from carrot or parsnep

in its chemical constitution, and contains one-twelfth of its weight of sugar, resembling that of the sugar cane.

ALKANET

Anchusa tinctoria

Class and Order, PENTANDRIA MONOGYNIA. NAT. ORD. BORAGINEÆ.
Gen. Char. *Calix* five-cleft; *Corolla* funnel-shaped; *Tube* strait, its mouth closed with convex, connivent scales; *Nuts* concave at the base.

ROOT perennial, long, externally of a purplish red colour; stems thick, round, branched, from one to two feet high; leaves long, linear, obtuse, partially surrounding the stem, the flowers varying as they advance in age from a red to a purple colour, thickly set together at the extremity of the branches; the stalks, leaves, and calices clothed with numerous rigid hairs.

Alkanet is not used medicinally; it is retained as an article of the Materia Medica, from the property it possesses of imparting a fine red colour to oils and fats.

COMMON CENTAURY

Erythræa centaurium

Class and Order, PENTANDRIA MONOGYNIA. NAT. ORD. GENTIANEÆ.
Gen. Char. *Calix* five cleft; *Corolla* funnel-shaped, continuing; *Limb* short; *Anthers* at length spirally twisted; *Style* erect; *Stigmas* two; *Capsule* linear, two-celled.—*Brown.*

ROOT annual, fibrous, woody; stalk from a few inches to a foot high or more, upright, smooth, and angular; leaves opposite, sessile, smooth, oblong, blunt at the point, and narrowed at the base; those of the stalk narrow, pointed, upright, three-ribbed, the uppermost often bent inwards; flowers rose-coloured, growing in a corymb, upright, and sessile; corolla monopetalous, funnel-shaped, the tube cylindrical, striated, extremely thin, twice the length of the calix; limb divided into five short ovate and spreading segments; stamens five; filaments white, thread-shaped, springing from the top of the tube; anthers oblong, incumbent, of a yellow colour, finally twisted; germen oblong, filling the tube of the corolla.

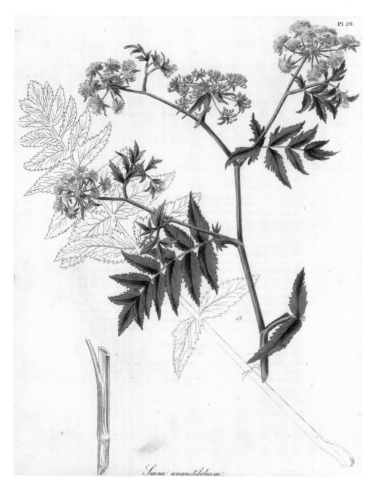

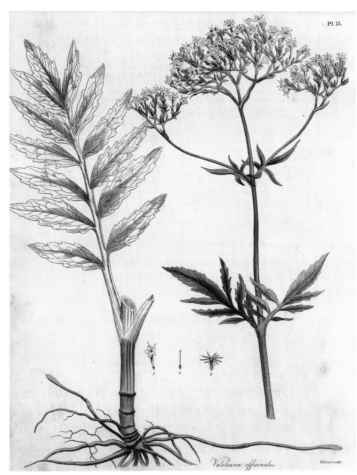

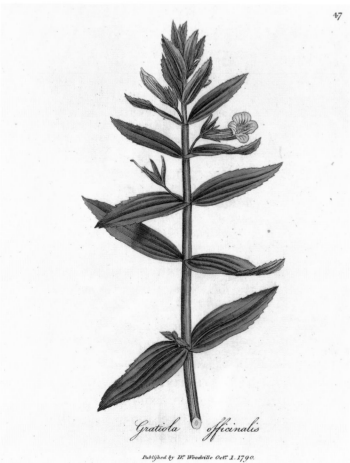

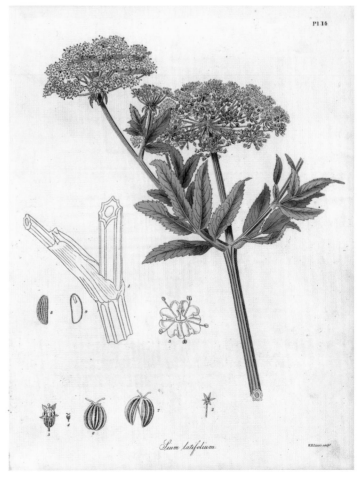

TOP LEFT: NARROW-LEAVED WATER PARSNEP, TOP RIGHT: WILD VALERIAN,
BOTTOM LEFT: HEDGE HYSSOP, BOTTOM RIGHT: BROAD-LEAVED WATER-PARSNEP

The variety of situations in which this plant grows in its wild state, appears to me to have occasioned the different appearances it assumes; on dry, chalky, and barren spots, in hedge-rows, and sometimes in woods, it assumes that form under which it is the *E. centaurium*; on sandy spots on the sea shore, it varies from an inch to four or five inches high, with its stem much branched; it is then *E. pulchella* or *littoralis*, and the broad-leaved variety, though appearing more like a species, may be found gradually emerging into one or other of the varieties.

I have repeatedly met with specimens having purely white flowers, but differing in no other respect from the common species. From its unpleasant, extremely bitter taste, it was known to the ancients by the appellation of *Fel teriæ* or Gall of the Earth; it was formerly in much repute, but it has given place to more powerful and less offensive bitters.

The *Erythræa centaurea*, like others of the Gentianeæ, contains a pure bitter, which is of value as a tonic; the leaves, young shoots, and flowers, are all active, and their bitterness is rendered more intense by drying. It has, as well as others of the same natural family, been given in intermittents, but its success is very dubious. M. Dulong d'Astafort has isolated the active principle of this plant, and has proposed giving it the name of *Centaurine*.

BISTORT OR SNAKEWEED

Polygonum bistorta

Class and Order, Octandria Trigynia. Nat. Ord. Polygoneæ.

Gen. Char. *Perianth* single, in five deep coloured, persistent segments, inferior; *Stamens* five to eight; *Styles* two or three; *Fruit* a one-seeded, compressed, or trigonous nut.

Root thick, with numerous small fibres, stems from one to two feet high; upper leaves with long sheaths; spikes cylindrical, very dense; flowers varying from a bright red to a pale pink or white-colour; stamens eight; styles three.

The Bistort is found in moist meadows in various parts of the kingdom, growing in large crowded patches; it is frequently cultivated in gardens, and increases rapidly by its roots; was formerly in repute for its styptic properties, but has now nearly fallen into disuse.

Sixty-eight species are enumerated.

The fresh root of the Bistort is astringent, and slightly acrid to the taste; it is tonic and astringent, and is useful in chronic diarrhœas, hæmorrhages, leucorrhœa, etc. Before the introduction of Cinchona, this, and many other indigenous tonics were given for the cure of intermittents; since the virtues of that remedy have become generally known, they have been entirely thrown aside. Bistort is generally administered in the form of powder; when combined with Gentian, the efficacy of both is said to be much increased. A decoction made by boiling two or three drachms of the fresh root with a pint of water, is frequently used as an injection in chronic ulceration of the vagina, urethra, and uterus. The poorer classes in Siberia eat the root, after its bitterness and astringency have been removed by water. Scheele has found oxalic acid in the root, which also contains a considerable quantity of fecula, on which its nutritious properties depend; a large proportion of tannin, and also of gallic acid.

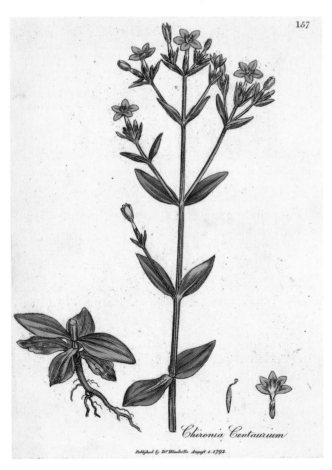

Chironia Centaurium

Published by Dr Woodville August 1 1792.

COMMON CENTAURY

The *P. hydropiper* has an acrid burning taste, which, like that of the *Arum maculatum*, is easily destroyed by heat; when applied to the skin it inflames it, and is occasionally used as a rubefacient in gouty affection.

P. fagopyrum is a native of Asia, but is naturalized in Europe. In Russia and some parts of Siberia this and the *P. tartaricum* form a large proportion of the food of the inhabitants. In France, the former is considered very valuable to the agriculturist, from the rapidity with which it ripens; in this country, it is also cultivated, and is known by the name of "Buckwheat." The seeds and root are both used in the northern parts of Europe, but in France and Britain the seeds only.

ANNUAL CAPSICUM OR GUINEA PEPPER

Capsicum annuum

Class and Order, PENTANDRIA MONOGYNIA. NAT. ORD. SOLANEÆ.
Gen. Char. *Corolla* rotate; *Berry* juiceless, with two cells.

ROOT annual; stem branched, angular, smooth, from one to two feet high; leaves ovate, pointed, smooth; flowers solitary, growing from the axils of the leaves, white, on longish petioles; fruit irregular in form, generally green at the base, and changing to a deep scarlet, orange, or yellow to the apex, inflated, either long or roundish, containing a dry spongy white pulp, with numerous flat kidney-shaped seeds.

The common capsicum is a native of both the Indies. It is of easy cultivation; requiring to be raised on a hot-bed, and, when the seedlings have attained a few inches in height, to be planted in the open border, where they will flower in June and July, and ripen their fruit in August, September, or later. All the species possess the pungent property of the common kind, but in greater or less excess.

The fruit of various species of capsicum is used as a condiment, under the name of Cayenne pepper. The *Capsicum annuum* is cultivated in Britain for the purpose of pickling; its fruit is used for this purpose, both in a green and ripe

state, but it never acquires that pungency for which the East and West India pickles are so much valued. The *Capsicum frutescens* is the hottest variety, and from it alone, the Cayenne pepper ought to be prepared.

The taste of Cayenne is pungent, and acrid, with a flavour peculiar to itself, and not capable of being classed either under the spicy or aromatic. In medicine, Cayenne is used internally in flatulence, and in cholera. In the latter, it seems to be useful; and, from my own experience, I would recommend it as an adjunct to other remedies, as it seems to allay to a great extent the nausea and retching, which are so distressing. In the form of gargle, it is found useful, in *Cynanche maligna*; as an external application to paralytic limbs; as an addition to sinapisms, to increase their rapidity and certainty; and in tropical fevers, where there is much determination to the head, as a substitute for Cantharides. Cayenne is said to stimulate the stomach alone, without causing the constitutional excitement, which most other spices occasion.

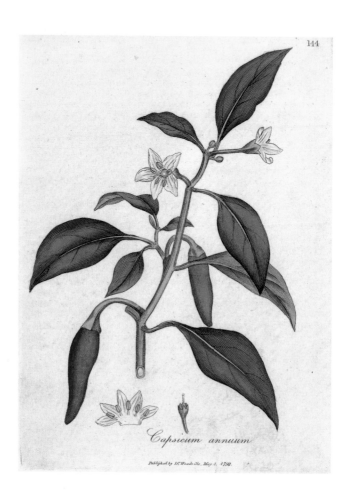

Capsicum annuum

GUINEA PEPPER OR ANNUAL CAPSICUM

SERRATED-LEAVED BOSWELLIA

Boswellia serrata

Class and Order, DECANDRIA MONOGYNIA. NAT. ORD. BURSERIACEÆ.
Gen. Char. *Calix* five-toothed, permanent; *Petals* five, obovate, oblong, spreading, with the margins incumbent in æstivation; *Disk* cup-shaped, crenated, staminiferous; *Stamens* ten; *Style* crowned by a capitate stigma; *Capsule* trigonal, three-valved, and three-celled; *Seed* solitary in the cells, girded by a *membrane.—Don.*

FROM Dr Roxburgh we learn, that the *Boswellia serrata*, or frankincense tree, is a native of the mountainous parts of Coromandel, attaining to a large size, and producing the drug known by the name of Olibanum. In the *Flora Indica*, Willdenow's *Canarium hirsutum* is regarded as this species, but this synonym is applied to another species, the *B. hirsuta*, by Sprengel, which has entire leaves. He describes three species, all of which produce a similar substance with that of the present plant.

Linnæus supposed olibanum to be the produce of the *Juniperus lycia*, but the researches of Dr Roxburgh and Mr Colebrooke have proved, that it is obtained from the *Boswellia serrata*, or *Libanus thurifera*.

Olibanum occurs in the form of semitransparent tears, of a pinkish colour, brittle when cold, but becoming unctuous when heated. Its taste is bitterish, pungent, and slightly aromatic. It burns with a clear steady flame, and diffuses an agreeable odour, and is used as incense in the ceremonials of the Greek and Roman Catholic churches. Olibanum was formerly used in affections of the chest. It is stimulant and diaphoretic, and is given by the native practitioners of India for the cure of gonorrhœa. It is also employed in rheumatism in the form of vapour.

GARDEN ANGELICA

Angelica archangelica

Class and Order, PENTANDRIA DIGYNIA. NAT. ORD. UMBELLIFERÆ.
Gen. Char. *Calix* obsolete; *Petals* elliptical, lanceolate, entire, and inflexed at the point; *Fruit* subcompressed, two winged; *Carpels* with three elevated dorsal ridges, the lateral ones spreading into the broad wings of the fruit; *Vittæ* various; *Universal involucre* scarcely any.

ANGELICA has most probably become naturalized to England, but it is rare in a wild state. Though commonly cultivated in gardens, it usually affects wet situations, but its aromatic property is more powerful when growing in dry places. The root is biennial, thick, and, in a young state, succulent, becoming woody as it advances in age; stems from three to six feet high, round, channelled, smooth, hollow, from one to two inches in diameter; leaves large, numerous, bipinnate; flowers in large umbels of a greenish-white, almost a pale sulphur colour.

This is probably the best of our native aromatics; it has a powerful smell,—to many too much so, to be agreeable, whilst to others it is a peculiar favourite. In England, its root is preserved with sugar, and sold as a confection for pectoral complaints.

Though not much used in modern practice, the *Angelica archangelica* is an excellent aromatic tonic. The whole plant has a pleasant aromatic odour, and a sweetish, rather acrid, aromatic taste. The root is the most active part, and, when wounded early in the spring, yields a small quantity of resinous juice, which becomes concrete when exposed to the air. If the root be dug up at this season and dried, the substance of it will be found intersected by numerous veins of this juice in a solid form.

The seeds are also active, and are occasionally employed as carminatives. The smaller stems, preserved with sugar, are used as stomachics, in the milder forms of dyspepsia, and as expectorants, in colds and slight pectoral affections.

CORIANDER

Coriandrum sativum

Class and Order, PENTANDRIA DIGYNIA. NAT. ORD. UMBELLIFERÆ.
Gen. Char. *Calix* of five teeth; *Petals* obcordate, point inflexed, outer one radiant, bifid; *Fruit* globose; *Carpels* with five primary ridges, depressed and wavy, of which the two lateral ones are placed in front of an accessary margin to the inner face; the four secondary ridges more prominent and carinated; *Interstices* without *vittæ*, the inner face of the carpel having two vittæ; *Seed* hollowed in front, covered by a loose membrane; *Universal Involucre* wanting; *Partial* on one side; *Carpels* adhering, separated with difficulty.—*Hooker.*

AN annual of easy culture, and found wild in some parts. This, which Dr Hooker says is the

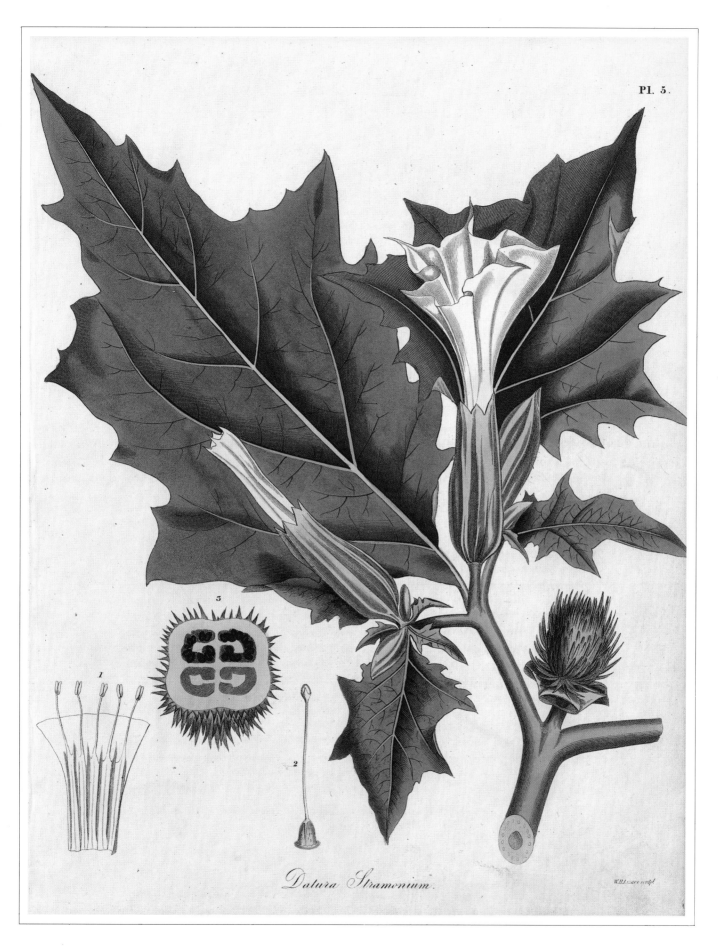

Pl. 5.

Datura Stramonium.

W.P.J. care sculpt

THORN-APPLE; FIG.1, A PORTION OF THE COROLLA LAID OPEN, SHOWING THE
INSERTION OF THE STAMENS; FIG.2, GERMEN AND PISTIL; FIG.3, TRANSVERSE
SECTION OF THE CAPSULE

only true species of the genus, has a long taper root; an erect leafy stem; bipinnate leaves; the pinnæ with broad wedge-shaped, toothed segments; the upper leaves becoming gradually more compressed, with very narrow linear segments; those of the upper ones almost setaceous; fruit hemispherical.

Like the Caraway, this plant, from long cultivation, has got dispersed, and is occasionally found wild amongst rubbish or neglected places; it is a native of Italy and the warm parts of Europe. Its seeds are much in request for confectionary as well as for medical uses; the whole plant has, in a fresh state, a powerful offensive smell, from which circumstance it acquires its name, κσζς, a bug. This it loses on drying, and then acquires an agreeable aromatic smell.

Coriander seeds are extensively employed as aromatic, carminative tonics. They contain an essential oil of a warm aromatic taste and pleasant smell. When fresh, the whole plant has a disagreeable odour, but when dried, the smell becomes grateful and aromatic. Like the seeds of the *Carum carui*, they are enveloped in sugar, and, like them, used as sweetmeats. They are frequently added to purgative infusions,— particularly to that of senna, to prevent tormina.

COMMON CARAWAY

Carum carui

Class and Order, Pentandria Digynia. Nat. Ord. Umbelliferæ.
Gen. Char. *Calix* obsolete; *Petals* obcordate; *Fruit* laterally compressed, oblong; *Carpels* with five filiform equal ridges, their inner faces plane; *Interstices* with single *vittæ*; *Seed* tereti-convex, plane in the front; *Universal and Partial Involucres* various.—*Hooker.*

This well-known plant is, and has long been, extensively cultivated, and most probably has so become naturalized to Britain. It grows naturally in the north of Europe. Its root is long and tapering; stem about two feet high, erect, branched, smooth, leafy, and deeply channelled; leaves, on the lower part of the stem on long foot-stalks, of a lively green, in appearance nearly resembling those of the carrot; such as grow on the upper parts of the stem are linear, narrow, opposite; one of them grows from a membranous-edged footstalk, the other small and nearly sessile; flowers growing in dense umbels. The caraway is cultivated for its seeds,

which are much used for medical and culinary purposes. In Scotland, the common name is *Carvey*, being slightly altered from the French and Italian, who call it Carvi.

The seeds of the *Carum carui* are, like those of many other umbelliferous plants, aromatic and stimulant. They are, perhaps, the most commonly used of any, and are excellent carminatives. Their taste, smell, and medical properties depend upon an essential oil, which they contain in large quantity, (about ¹⁄₂₀th of their weight.) The taste of both is warm, pungent, and aromatic.

In colic and gastrodynia, a few drops of this oil, or half a teaspoonful of the seeds, are sovereign remedies. Richard recommends that a liniment, formed by adding a few drops of this oil to a small quantity of olive oil, be rubbed over the pit of the stomach or the abdomen, in cases of colic.

Caraway seeds are frequently added to bread and biscuit, both for the flavour which they impart, and for the purpose of aiding digestion. Enveloped in sugar, they are much used as sweetmeats. The roots of the Carum are aromatic, and when boiled, are said to be pleasant substitutes for parsneps.

COMMON DILL

Anethum graveolens

Class and Order, Pentandria Digynia. Nat. Ord. Umbelliferæ.
Gen. Char. *Carpels* elliptic oblong, compressed, with five equidistant ridges; *Petals* obovate, inflexed, entire.

Root biennial long, whitish, producing two or three stems, which are upright, smooth, deeply channelled, branched, about two feet high; leaves on sheathing footstalks, growing from the joints of the stalks, alternate, smooth, doubly pinnate, the pinnæ linear and pointed; flowers in terminal umbels, yellow, the petals inflexed at the tips.

Dill is a native of Spain and Portugal, but has been cultivated in English gardens since the time of Gerard, 1597. Its seeds are warm and aromatic, like most others of the Umbelliferæ, but possess no peculiar virtue that is not found more abundantly and of a more agreeable flavour in others of the family.

The seeds of the *Anethum graveolens* have a

strong disagreeable odour, and a warm, somewhat aromatic taste. They owe their activity to a volatile oil, which they contain in considerable quantity, and are powerfully stimulating, but as there are so many more pleasant stimuli possessed of equal medicinal virtues, they are not often prescribed. The distilled water is prepared from the seeds; a pound of these are to be bruised and distilled with a sufficient quantity of water to prevent empyreuma, and the process is to be stopped when about a gallon has passed over. Nearly half an ounce of volatile oil is procured from a pound of the seeds.

Dr Ainslie states that the dill seeds are a favourite remedy among the native practitioners of India, and that they seldom fail in curing the flatulent colic of young children.

HEMLOCK WATER-PARSNEP

Œnanthe crocata

Class and Order, Pentandria Digynia. Nat. Ord. Umbelliferæ.
Gen. Char. *Calix* of five teeth; *Petals* obcordate, with an inflexed point; *Fruit* subterete, crowned with the short styles; *Carpels* with five blunt convex ridges, of which the lateral ones are marginal and a little broader; *Interstices* with single *vittæ*; *Seed* tereti-convex, Axis none; *Universal involucre* various; *Partial* of many leaves; *Flowers* of the ray on long pedicles, sterile; those of the *Disk* sessile or shortly pediculate, fertile.—*Hooker.*

Root composed of numerous tubers, resembling small parsneps, of a whitish colour; stems two or three feet high, branched, hollow, deeply furrowed, the angles acute; leaves long, smooth and shining. The whole plant abounds in a yellow juice of a poisonous quality, and is one of the most virulent poisons among our native plants; six species are British, all of which are of a suspicious nature; frequent accidents have occurred from their inadvertent use. The present species is met with in wet pastures by the sides of ditches, and is said to be particularly injurious, "to brood mares that sometimes eat the root." I should suspect there is some error in this, as the roots are situated quite beneath the soil; but as the whole plant abounds with a fœtid juice, it is likely to have been consumed with other herbage, and to have injured horses as well as other animals.

Dr Christison, speaking of the Œnanthe crocata, says "It seems to be the most energetic of the umbelliferous vegetables. In none of the fatal cases was life prolonged beyond three hours and a-half, and in several, death took place within an hour. One man was killed by a single spoonful of the juice." Orfila gives a minute account of several fatal cases of poisoning with the root of this plant. The symptoms caused in man, are nausea, vertigo, intense pain in the stomach and bowels, diarrhœa, burning heat of the mouth and throat, tetanic convulsions, coma, delirium, and occasionally discharge of blood from the mouth and nose. After death, the stomach and intestines are found of a reddish purple colour, with gangrenous patches dispersed on their surface. From the symptoms and morbid appearances, Orfila draws the conclusion, that it acts as an energetic local irritant; and that it also acts violently on the nervous system. In cases of poisoning with the Œnanthe, the instantaneous evacuation of the stomach by emetics is to be attempted, blood-letting is to be had recourse to, and mucilaginous drinks are to be administered. After the immediate danger from the narcotic action of the poison is over, the acrid effects are to be combated by the application of leeches and blisters, to the epigastrium and abdomen; and if

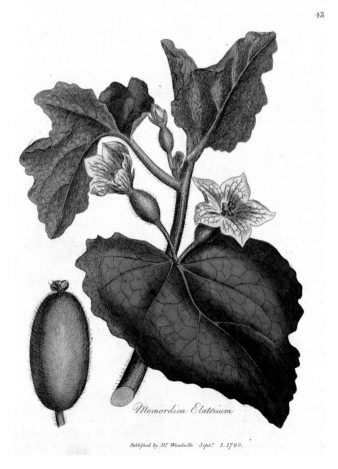

Momordica Elaterium

Published by Dr Woodville Sept.ʳ 1. 1790.

WILD OR SPIRTING CUCUMBER

delirium continue, cold to the head, and cupping, or other antiphlogistic measures, are to be employed.

The same plan of treatment applies to the Cicuta, Æthusa, and others of the same class of poisons. This plant is not used in medicine, but the bruised root is frequently employed by the people of Brittany, as an external application to hæmorrhoids. It is a very dangerous remedy.

FŒTID HELLEBORE OR BEARSFOOT

Helleborus fœtidus

Class and Order, POLYANDRIA POLYGYNIA. NAT. ORD. RANUNCULACEÆ.
TRIBE IV.—HELLEBOREÆ.
Gen. Char. *Calix* of five persistent leaves; *Petals* eight or ten, small, tubular, two-lipped, nectariferous; *Pericarps* or *Follicles* nearly erect, many-seeded.

A hardy perennial, growing in many parts of Great Britain, in clayey and calcareous soils; but it is to be suspected that it has become naturalized, being formerly much cultivated as a domestic medicine, particularly as a vermifuge.

The root is fibrous, and descends deep into the soil; stem from a foot and a-half to two feet high, leafy; leaves on long, deeply-channelled footstalks, which nearly surround the stem; the lower leaves divided into five, seven, or nine leaflets, thick, almost coriaceous, in substance, serrated, of a very dark-green. As the leaves ascend the stem, they become more entire, and the upper ones assume the character of bracteas, being of an unusually bright pale-yellow green; flowers numerous, of a green colour; tips of the petals purplish; the whole plant powerfully fœtid.

The fœtid hellebore is possessed of similar properties with the other species, and Curtis remarked many years ago, that a very innocent fraud was constantly practised, in substituting the roots of the fœtid and green hellebores for those of the black, *H. niger*: but as their properties appear identical, no inconvenience arises from the substituting of the one for the other. Ten species are enumerated in Don's System of Gardening, natives of various parts of Europe.

The leaves of the *Helleborus fœtidus* have an acrid, bitter, and nauseous taste; they are occasionally employed as a domestic vermifuge; but

as fatal effects have sometimes followed their incautious exhibition, their use is attended with danger. The *Helleborus fœtidus* is said by Dr Christison, on the authority of Buchner, to be the most poisonous of the genus.

I have not met with any good analysis of the *H. fœtidus*; the medical and poisonous properties of this genus, and their chemical constitution, will be considered under the article *H. niger*.

FLY AMANITA

Amanita muscaria

Class and Order, CRYPTOGAMIA FUNGI. NAT. ORD. FUNGI.
Gen. Char. Bursting from a *volva*; *Pileus* fleshy, generally warted; *Gills* crowded, nearly entire; *Stipes* mostly elongated, annulate or naked.

THIS elegant species is diffused widely, growing on banks, shady woods, and occasionally in open plains, sheep walks, or in damp meadows. The variety of places in which it grows, does not seem to induce the variations in colour, as it may be found growing in the same places of all shades, from cream-colour to the most intense and brilliant scarlet, sometimes coated as it were, with thick varnish, and at other times quite opaque; in rapidity of growth but few of this tribe exceed it. Some years ago, I gathered a beautiful specimen, in the month of October, the pileus was about three inches in diameter. Not having a box with me, I put it into the crown of my hat, where it continued some hours. On my return home I removed it from the hat, and found it had expanded so much, as to be nearly of the diameter of the hat, and the stem, which had so far accommodated itself to circumstances, not being able to elongate, spread laterally so as to form a broad flat stipes. The present, which I cannot but esteem specifically distinct from the following species, (*A. verrucosa*,) is of much larger size, and never, as far as I have seen, assumes a green colour, as that often does; the taste of both is alike, being exceedingly pungent. Though the *muscaria* is used for the purpose of destroying flies, it is eaten by a variety of other insects. I have repeatedly eaten small quantities of the *muscaria* and *verrucosa*, and have always experienced the same effects from both; a burning sensation at the back of the throat, almost insupportable for a short

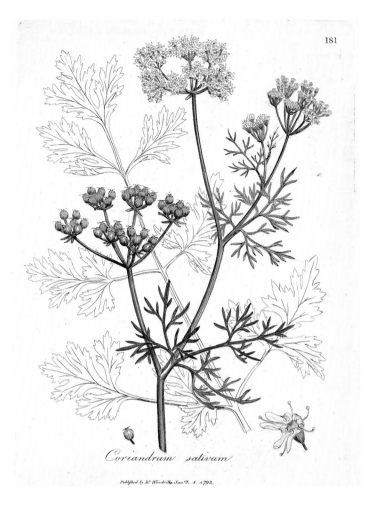

Coriandrum sativum

Published by Dʳ Woodville Janᵧ 1. 1793.

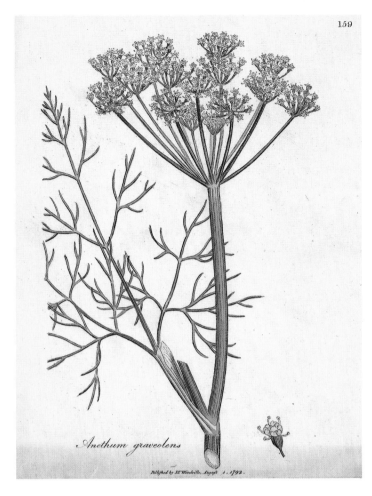

Anethum graveolens

Published by Dʳ Woodville August 1. 1792.

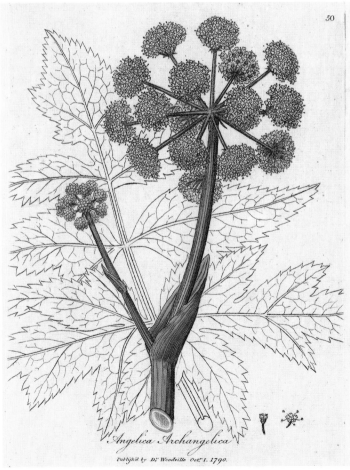

Angelica Archangelica

Published by Dʳ Woodville Octᵣ 1. 1790.

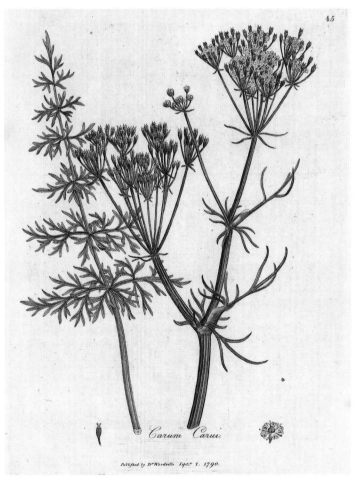

Carum Carui

Published by Dʳ Woodville Septᵣ 1. 1790.

TOP LEFT: CORIANDER, TOP RIGHT: COMMON DILL, BOTTOM LEFT: GARDEN
ANGELICA, BOTTOM RIGHT: COMMON CARAWAY

time, but much relieved by drinking milk, though the peculiar sense of burning continued for six or eight hours.

The accompanying figures of *A. verrucosa* will suffice to point out the species; its places of growth, and effects when eaten being precisely those of *A. muscaria*, further description appears unnecessary.

Numerous fatal accidents occur on the Continent, from the *Amanita muscaria* being eaten instead of the *A. cæsarea*, to which it bears a great resemblance. The following account is quoted by Orfila, from the Inaugural Dissertation of M. Vadrot.

Several French soldiers, near Polosk in Russia, ate a quantity of the *Amanita muscaria*, which they had mistaken for the *A. cæsarea*; four of them, men of strong constitutions, believed themselves safe from the bad effects which had already shown themselves in their companions, and therefore refused to take emetics. In the evening, however, the following symptoms set in; anxiety, sense of suffocation, burning thirst, severe griping pains; the pulse became small and irregular, and the body covered with a cold sweat, the lineaments of the countenance were changed in a remarkable manner, the nose and lips acquired a violet hue;

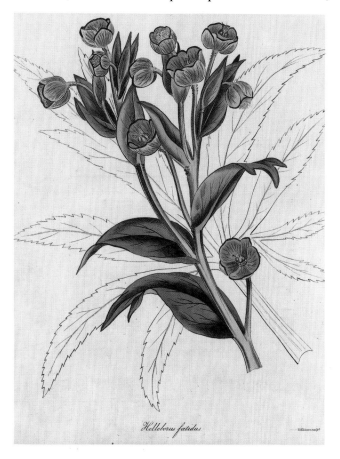

Helleborus fœtidus

FOETID HELLEBORE OR BEARSFOOT

violent tremblings came on, the abdomen swelled, and a profuse fœtid diarrhœa supervened.

These symptoms increased in violence, and the men were conveyed to the hospital; the extremities became cold and livid, they suffered excruciating pain, and were delirious; one died soon after his admission to the hospital; and the other three, before morning. On dissection, the stomach and intestines were found inflated by fœtid gas, their inner surfaces exhibited marks of inflammation, and there were numerous gangrenous patches; the liver was much swelled, and the gall-bladder filled with dark thick bile. Several of the comrades of these soldiers, who had submitted at first to medical treatment, recovered, after much suffering.

Most of the poisonous fungi belong to the narcotico-acrid section of poisons, so that in the majority of cases, narcotism and violent irritation will probably be combined; in the above account symptoms of irritant poisoning preponderate. In a case mentioned by Dr Christison, where a man eat a large quantity of *Agaricus campanulatus*, pure narcotism was the result, and before he had concluded his repast he was seized with dimness of sight, giddiness, trembling, and loss of recollection. He recovered so far as to be able to go in search of assistance, but before he had proceeded 250 yards, his memory again failed him, and he lost his way. His countenance expressed anxiety, his pulse was slow and weak, he reeled and could not articulate. He became so drowsy that he could be kept awake only by constant dragging. Vomiting was produced by sulphate of zinc, and the drowsiness gradually went off. Next day he complained only of languor and weakness.

The *Amanita muscaria* though so poisonous in France and most parts of Europe, is used in Kamtschatka and northern Russia, for producing intoxication. Its effects are similar to those produced by opium, the person feels happy, speaks and moves involuntarily. Its effects are often ludicrous; if a person completely under its influence wish to step over a straw, he takes a stride of sufficient extent, to clear the trunk of a tree; a talkative person cannot keep silence or secrets; and a musical person is constantly singing.

In Germany Dr Reinhard has used the *A. muscaria* with success in paralysis, epilepsy, and in chronic catarrh, where there is muco-purulent expectoration. M. Paulet has also employed it as an application to cancerous and ill-conditioned ulcers.

Murray, in his Apparatus Medicaminum has mentioned that benefit is to be derived from the use of this remedy in diseases of the skin, scirrhous tumours, and in epilepsy.

GLUTINOUS AGARIC

Agaricus semiglobatus

Class and Order, Cryptogamia Fungi. Nat. Ord. Fungi. Gen. Char. *Volva* none; *Pileus* with gills beneath, differing in substance from the rest of the plant.

Much ambiguity exists with regard to the properties of the present species, and I have little doubt but that much of the difference of opinion is occasioned by the circumstances of soil and situation in which the specimens grow. I ate several gathered from the spot where those were procured which proved fatal to the family at Mitcham, only two or three days after the occurrence, as detailed by Mr Parrot in the London Med. and Phys. Journal, v. xx. without experiencing any other effect, than a slight burning sensation in the throat, and others had no other taste than what is common to our best mushrooms. My deceased relative, the late Mr Curtis, was a curious and close observer of this tribe of vegetables, and I regret his name of *glutinosous* has been changed, on account of the frequent inapplicability of the present name to the species, and his name being more likely to identify it. Much stress has been laid upon the globular or acuminated form of the pileus. Of this I can speak confidently, that a specimen with an acuminated pileus will often become flattened in the course of a day, and that I should rather depend upon the glutinous cap and stem, then to any character drawn from the shape; as in this tribe of plants their mode of growth and forms they assume, often depend upon casual circumstances, as a stone or other extraneous substance lying in their way, they will sometimes grow round it, or, if growing up between two stones, the shape they assume is that of the interstice from which they spring.

This species varies in size from half an inch to two inches in diameter, and from one to four or five inches in height; its usual colour is a dull dirty yellow-brown, becoming darker when moist; it is more gradual in decay than many others, and though it shrinks much, may be dried between paper like other plants.

It is an abundant species, growing in moist pastures, and often in great abundance, mostly singly, but occasionally in clusters; there is nothing acrimonius or disagreeable in its general taste, yet its appearance will not recommend it to the lovers of mushrooms; and I cannot but doubt whether the fatal effects ascribed to this, do not belong to some other species.

The poisonous properties of *Agaricus semiglobatus* are not well ascertained; Mr Sowerby in the London Med. and Physical Journal, classes it among the poisonous fungi. Of its chemical or medicinal properties nothing is known.

WILD OR SPIRTING CUCUMBER

Momordica elaterium

Class and Order, Monœcia Monadelphia. Nat. Ord. Cucurbitaceæ. Gen. Char. Male. *Calix* five-cleft; *Corolla* five-parted; *Filaments* five. **Female.** *Calix* five-cleft; *Corolla* five-parted; *Style* trifid; *Fruit* opening elastically.

This species is a native of the south of Europe, and is cultivated on account of its medical properties. It forms a low trailing vine; its root is annual, long, and fleshy; stems several, round, branching, thick, and rough, with coarse hairs, without tendrils; leaves on long footstalks, irregularly heart-shaped, sinuated, veined, the upper surface a deep green, paler beneath; flowers of both sexes growing in clusters; the male flowers on short footstalks, the female sessile on the germen; the whole plant beset with bristly hairs.

The cultivation of this plant is similar to that of the common cucumber, it is equally hardy, and readily produces its fruit, without requiring shelter except in the seedling-state. The seeds should be raised on a hot-bed, and planted out early in the spring; they flower during the summer months, and produce ripe fruit in August and September, and sometimes later. The plants are very susceptible of cold, and are usually destroyed the first sharp frost. It derives its name of squirting or spirting cucumber, from the fruit detaching itself on the slightest touch from the footstalks, and discharging the seeds and pulp through the aperture where the footstalk was inserted.

Elaterium is prepared by slicing the fresh fruit of the Momordica, and allowing the juice which exudes to remain for some time in an earthen vessel; the sediment which is deposited, is to be collected on a piece of fine linen, and gently dried. Dr Clutterbuck gives an excellent account of the mode of preparing this drug. It is called an *Extract* in the London and Dublin Pharmacopœias, but it is not prepared as the other extracts are, and perhaps *Feculence* might be a more appropriate name for this, and other substances of a similar nature. The French prepare the extract by inspissating the filtered juice of the fresh fruit; thus the *Feculence*, the most active part, is thrown away. Elaterium, as prepared according to Dr Clutterbuck's process, occurs in small pieces of about the sixteenth of an inch in thickness, of a light greyish colour, porous, of a disagreeable smell, and of a bitter, mawkish, taste. In anascarca, much benefit is often derived from the use of this remedy; it causes copius watery evacuations from the bowels, and generally gives relief. It is not admissible where the patient is much reduced in strength, or where there is a tendency to diarrhœa.

The great uncertainty of the effects of Elaterium as a cathartic, and the probable dependence of this uncertainty on original differences in the quality of the drug, as well as on the occasional addition of impurities, render it an object of much consequence to determine what is its active principle, and how this may be separated in a pure state.

LONG-LEAVED WATER HEM-LOCK OR COWBANE

Cicuta virosa

Class and Order, Pentandria Digynia. Nat. Ord. Umbelliferæ.
Gen. Char. *Calix* of five teeth, leafy; *Petals* obcordate, with an inflexed point; *Fruit* in pairs, roundish, contracted at the sides; *Carpels* with five, nearly plain equal ridges, of which the lateral ones are marginal; *Interstices* with single *vittæ*, which in the dry fruit are more raised than the ridges; *Seed* round.—*Hooker.*

Root large, hollow and divided by transverse partitions into numerous cells; stalks three feet high, branched; leaves long, narrow, serrated, generally growing in threes, sometimes in pairs.

The form of the leaves and root differ from all the other British Umbelliferæ. It is not of very common occurrence, but is occasionally found throughout this kingdom. It is probably one of the most virulent poisons produced by the British Flora, its deleterious qualities have proved fatal to men and kine, but horses, sheep and goats are said not to be injured by it. Another species, *C. maculata*, has been used in medicine as the *Conium maculatum*.

Many fatal instances of poisoning with the *Cicuta virosa*, are on record. Orfila quotes from Wepfer the following case. "*Mœder*, six years of age, accompanied by a child of eight, and by six little girls, eat some of the roots of the *cicuta*, which he took for parsneps. Soon after he experienced great anxiety, uttered a few words, lay down and made water; shortly after he became horribly convulsed, lost the use of his senses, and closed his mouth firmly; he gnashed his teeth, rolled his eyes, and blood was observed to flow from his ears. He had frequent hiccup, and made efforts to vomit, but was unable to open his mouth; he had severe pain in his joints, his head was bent back, and the opisthotonos was so violent that a little child might have crept under the arch formed between his back and the bed. When the convulsions had ceased he implored his mother's assistance; but though all means were used to revive him, his strength rapidly diminished, and he died in half an hour after the invasion of the symptoms. The abdomen and face became swelled after death; a degree of lividity appeared round the eyes; and a quantity of green froth flowed from the mouth for a considerable time. Of the other children who had eaten this plant, the child of eight years of age, who had taken a considerable quantity, died; the other six recovered after having experienced severe symptoms."

Metzdorff has related the particulars of the inspection of three cases which have proved quickly fatal with convulsions and vomiting. Nothing remarkable seems to have been found except great gorging of the cerebral vessels.

The *Cicuta* is seldom used in medicine, but is said by some, to possess all the properties of the *Conium maculatum*, and to act with greater certainty in a smaller dose. Haller, and many other writers suppose this to have been the plant, by the juice of which Socrates was poisoned.

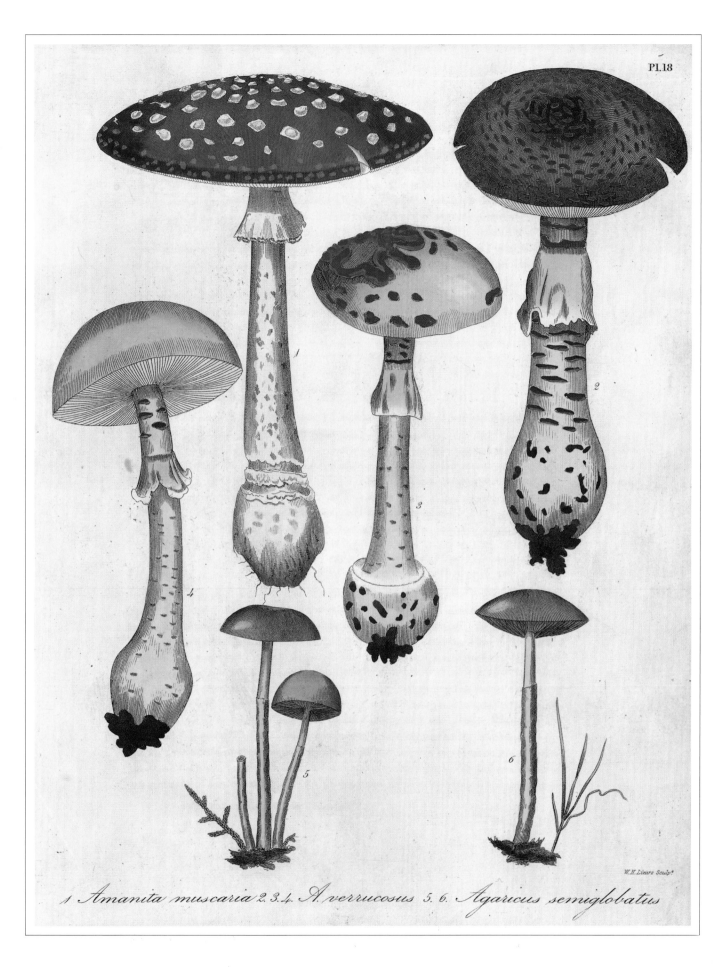

Pl.18

W.H.Lizars Sculp.

1 Amanita muscaria 2.3.4. A. verrucosus 5.6. Agaricus semiglobatus

FLY AMANITA AND GLUTINOUS AGARIC; FIG.1, AMANITA MUSCARIA; FIGS.2,3,4,
AMANITA VERRUCOSA; FIG.5,6, AGARICUS SEMI-GLOBATUS.

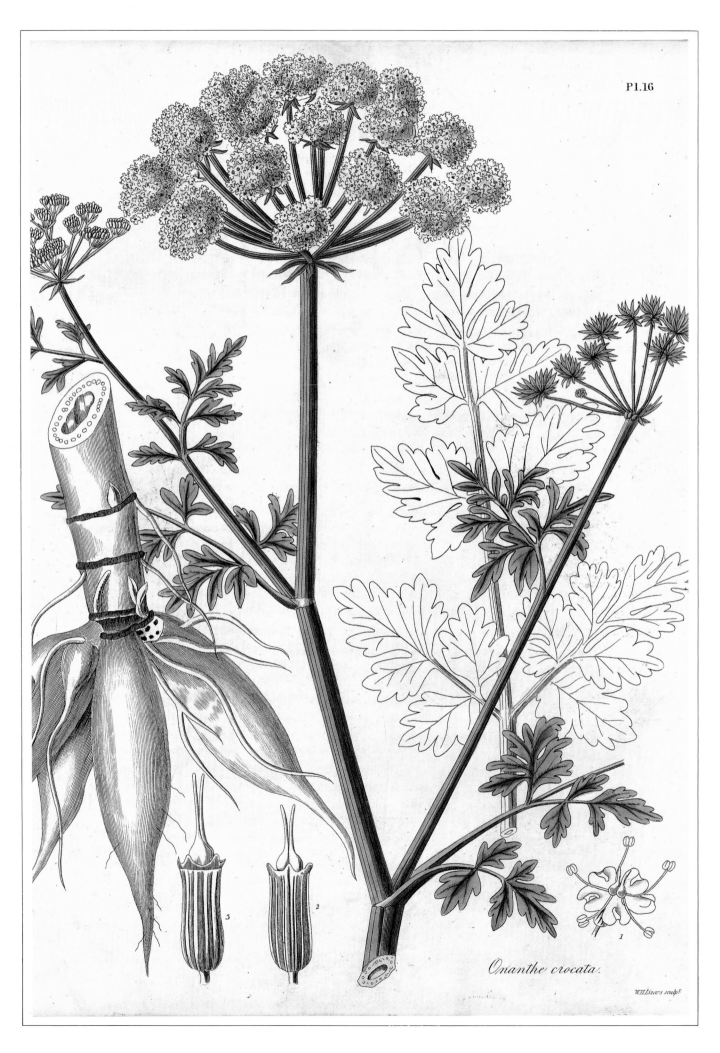

Onanthe crocata.

WH.Lizars sculp.

44   HEMLOCK WATER-PARSNEP; FIG.1, A FLOWER; FIG.2 AND 3, SEEDS. ALL MAGNIFIED.

SUGAR CANE

Saccharum officinarum

Class and Order, Triandria Digynia. Nat. Ord. Gramineæ.
Gen. Char. *Spikelets* in pairs, alternatively sessile and pedicelled, hermaphrodite, one-flowered; *Glumes* two, coriaceous; *Flowers* hermaphrodite, valves two, transparent, shining, the lower one notched, or awned, surrounded at the base with silky hairs.

Root perennial, solid, jointed; stems many, growing from the same root, rising to eight, twelve, or more feet high, upright, round, smooth, leafy, jointed; leaves long, embracing the stem; panicle loose, erect, or slightly inclining, about two feet in length, calix of three valves, one-flowered; flowers small, two-valved, beset at the base with long silky hairs.

The Sugar Cane is a plant of the utmost importance, not only in medicine, but for economical purposes, and is the staple produce of the British West India Islands. In the East Indies it is also cultivated, but in Dr Roxburgh's *Flora Indica*, he says that in 1796 a new species, *S. sinensis* was introduced from China, which promised considerable advantages over the *S. officinarum*, "particularly from its being so solid and hard, as to resist the forceps of the white ant, and the teeth of the jackal, two great enemies to East India sugar plantations. At the same time it bears the drought much better than the sorts in general cultivation, it produces a profitable crop even to the third year, while the common cane of India must be renewed every year; it is also said to yield juice of a richer quality."

Numerous plants of different families, produce sugar in greater or less quantity, and are accordingly cultivated in various countries for this substance. One of the most productive is the sugar maple of America, from which the sugar is obtained by wounding the tree and collecting the juice as it exudes, and evaporating it, and it may likewise be procured from the maple and sycamore of this country, but in small quantity, and inferior in quality; in France, carrot and beet-roots are cultivated for their saccharine juice; it is sometimes to be found in a crystalline form, and nearly pure, in the stems and roots of some of our native grasses; as the *Poa aquatica*, *Poa fluitans*, and *Catabrosa aquatica*. It is not a little remarkable that the British species of grass

in which sugar is found in a crystalline form, are entirely aquatic; I first met with it in this state in *Poa aquatica*. The circumstance which led me to discover it, was, observing some swine eagerly rooting among mud and weeds that were thrown out of a water course. I remarked they greedily devoured the roots and stems of some species of grass, which induced me to examine the kind, which proved to be those of the *Poa aquatica*. The roots were large and succulent, but having been exposed to the action of the sun and air for some days, the outer parts of the stems and roots had become dry. I peeled one or two of these, and at the base of each leaf, and of the sheaths covering the root, I found some small transparent crystals, which were pure sugar. I obtained nearly half an ounce of these, and have since found that this plant, as well as the other two above named, which are the sweetest of our native grasses, if removed from the watery spots in which they constantly grow, and exposed to the action of the sun and air, produce small grains of sugar as before-mentioned. Several species of Fucus or sea-weed, also spontaneously exude sugar. The farinaceous parts of grain are capable of being converted into sugar, as is observable in the process of malting; the barley is spread upon a floor, then wetted and thrown into a heap. When natural fermentation commences, the grain, by the action of the water and increased temperature, begins to vegetate, and is then speedily dried in a kiln, which converts the fecula of the seed into a saccharine substance.

Sugar is highly nutritious, and those plants in which it most abounds, as numerous species of the Gramineæ, the carrot, beet, &c. are those which afford the greatest portions of sustenance to man as well as the inferior animals.

The greater part of the sugar, which is consumed in Europe, is the produce of the *Saccharum officinarum*, and is imported from the West Indian Islands. A considerable quantity is also imported from the Mauritius, the Brazils, and the East Indies. Sugar is prepared thus;—To the fresh juice obtained by expression, a small quantity of quicklime is added, (about 1 part of lime to 800 of juice,) by this means, the free acid is saturated, and the mucilaginous and other impurities, which would impede the crystallization, separated. The juice thus treated, is then gradually boiled down to the proper consistence, and the impurities, which rise in the form of scum, removed. It is then cooled in shallow vessels. When cool it forms a soft mass, consisting of numerous small crystals, imbedded in a thick tenacious syrup, to free it from which it is put into casks, in the bottom of which holes are bored; through these the syrup gradually drains, and the sugar is left in the state called, *Raw* or *Brown sugar*. The syrup which drops, is used along with other refuse for making rum, and is, in its purest form, exported to Europe, where it is used for various domestic purposes. The refining of sugar is performed in Europe. The process is as follows;—The sugar to be refined, is dissolved in water heated by steam, it is then evaporated *in vacuo*, and put into moulds of a conical shape, with a hole in the apex; when the sugar has become solid, a small quantity of saturated syrup is poured on the base of the cone, this, in its passage to the apex, carries away any impurity which may be present, and is more economical than pure water, which was formerly employed; the latter part of the process, (that of washing the sugar with syrup,) is conducted in apartments heated to about 150°F. When dry, the sugar is removed from the moulds, and is sold as *Loaf* or *White sugar*. The evaporation *in vacuo*, and purification by saturated syrup, are modern improvements. A still further improvement has been lately suggested, and is at present under the consideration of Government. It is proposed, that the processes of crystallization and refining, shall be conducted in England, and that the juice shall only undergo boiling sufficient to allow of its being imported without undergoing fermentation.

During the war between Britain and France, when the produce of Britain's colonies was not allowed to enter hostile ports, the French and other continental nations employed the sugar of the Beet, *Beta vulgaris*, as a substitute for that of the cane; *Achard* was the first who tried it on a large scale, and though he to a certain extent succeeded, yet the sugar prepared could not compete with that of the colonies; since that period, however, the manufacture of beet sugar has arrived at such perfection, that it equals in all its properties that of the cane.

Most fruits, and many vegetables, contain sugar variously modified; in the process of germination, it is formed in considerable quantity. In America, the maple-sugar, prepared from the juice of the tree itself, is used as a substitute for the cane-sugar, but it has a peculiar flavour, and does not possess so great a sweetening power.

In the East Indies, the natives prepare a sort of sugar from the juice of various species of palm; the juice is called toddy; and when fermented, is used as an intoxicating liquor: the sugar is called Jaggery, and is supposed by the native practitioners to possess considerable medicinal virtues.

Sugar is not used in medicine in an uncombined form; but is extensively employed for the purpose of covering the nauseous taste of some drugs; for ameliorating the acrimony of others; and for rendering another class miscible with fluids, with which they were previously incompatible. It is the base of lozenges; and in the state of sugar-candy or barley-sugar, is useful in colds where there is much irritation of the upper part of the larynx.

Sugar may be divided into the following classes:

1. Cane Sugar: *a.* Sugar from the cane itself. *b.* Sugar from the maple. *c.* From the beet. *d.* From various grasses, *Holci, Poæ,* etc.

2. Grape Sugar. *a.* From grapes. *b.* From starch and vegetable matters by the action of sulphuric acid. *c.* From honey. *d.* That obtained from the urine of diabetic patients. *e.* Sugar of milk.

3. Sugar of Mushroom, discovered by Braconnot, and contained in many species of Fungi.

4. Liquid Sugar. Contained in an immense number of vegetables; we are familiar with it in the form of molasses or treacle, which most chemists look upon as deriving its sweetness, from liquid sugar contained in the juice of the cane, and not depending on the quantity of crystallized sugar which it contains. A sugar of this sort exists in honey.

5. Sugar from Manna. *a.* From manna itself, (Mannite.) *b.* From the leaves of various plants, celery, etc. *c.* From fermented honey. *d.* From fermented beet juice.

6. From the liquorice root. *a.* From *Glycyrrhiza glabra,* (Glycyrrhizine.) *b.* From the *Abrus precatorius. c.* From *Polypodium vulgare.*

Many other varieties might be enumerated, but these seem to me the principal.

Molasses or *Treacle* is the empyreumatic syrup which drains from the sugar during its first and subsequent crystallizations; it is of a

Pl. 19

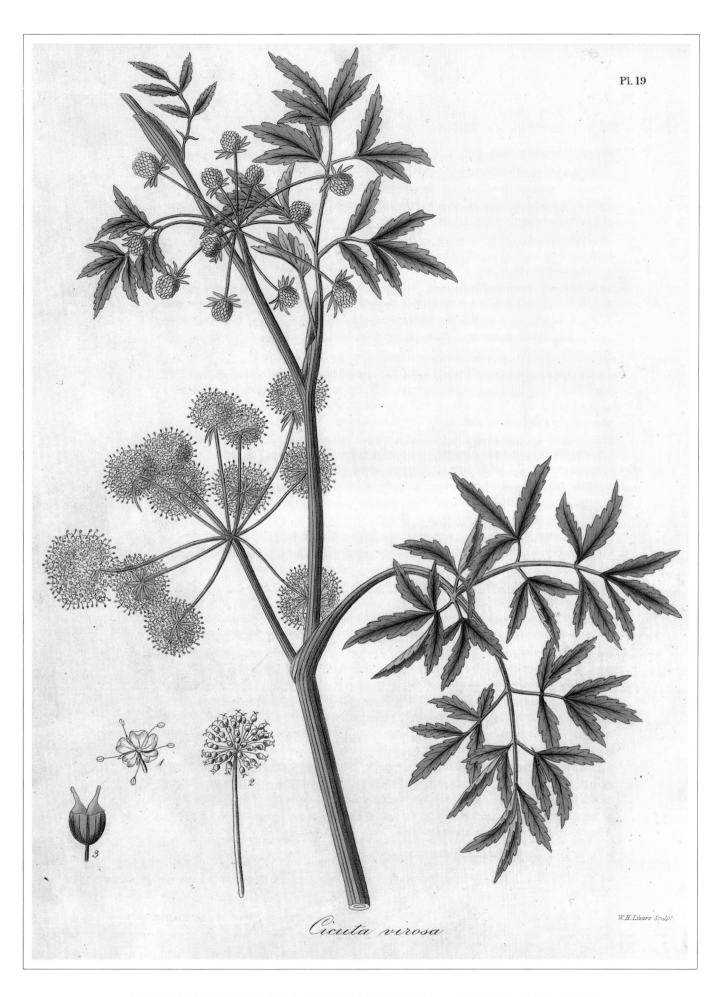

Cicuta virosa

W.H.Lizars Sculp.

LONG-LEAVED WATER HEMLOCK OR COWBANE; FIG.1, A FLOWER; FIG.2, AN UMBEL
WITH FRUIT; FIG.3, A SINGLE FRUIT; FIGS.1 AND 3 MAGNIFIED.

pleasant subacid sweet taste, and is extensively used for various domestic purposes. In pharmacy it is employed for making several syrups; it is in itself gently laxative, and expectorant, and is a common domestic remedy in the form of what is called a "treacle posset," in colds, febrile attacks, and many of the milder diseases of children.

IPECACUANHA

Cephaelis ipecacuanha

Class and Order, Pentandria Monogynia. Nat. Ord. Cinchonaceæ.
Gen. Char. *Calix* four-toothed; *Flowers* in a dense involucrated head; *Corolla* funnel-shaped; *Tube* hairy, limb five-parted; *Stamens* five, included; *Stigma* bifid; *Drupe* two-seeded.

THE Ipecacuan is a dwarf, almost herbaceous plant, with long straggling roots, or rather the stems are prostrate, and throw up occasionally a short stalk with a few rather large, oval, pointed leaves, the inflorescence terminal. From these creeping stems, grow two kinds of roots, one simply fibrous, the other knotty or granulated, growing either singly or in fasciculi. These latter do not appear to possess the power of reproduction, whilst cuttings from the stems that have fibrous roots attached, grow readily. It is a native of low damp woods and forests in Brazil, and was long unknown in this country, though the drug had been in use for more than two centuries.

A variety of plants are endued with emetic properties, but we are unacquainted with any one on which so much reliance can be placed as to its effect, as the Ipecacuan. This circumstance naturally creates a large demand, and subjects it to numerous adulterations, the most common of which is its mixture with some species of Ionidium, and occasionally with the roots of other plants. The true drug may be known by its colour and odour, particularly if moistened, likewise by its granulated form. The other roots which are known in the shops as the black or white ipecacuan, have the bark of their roots either only cracked, or sometimes with deep fissures, but not adhering in separate knots or joints as in the roots of the Cephaëlis, and a transverse section of each shows, as in the annexed figures, a difference in their internal structure. Ipecacuan, when good, should be

moderately dry, with a grey or ash-coloured bark, having a resinous appearance, both internally and externally; the substance of the roots should be a pale whitish brown, becoming darker when moistened, and giving out its peculiar odour. It is not so heavy as the roots of the Richardsonia, but heavier than either the Psychotria or Ionidium. The knotty parts of the roots are those possessed of the most active properties, and the fibrous ones should be rejected. Figure 1. on the annexed cut represents the officinal part of the plant; figure 2. a transverse section of the root, showing the cortical and woody parts.

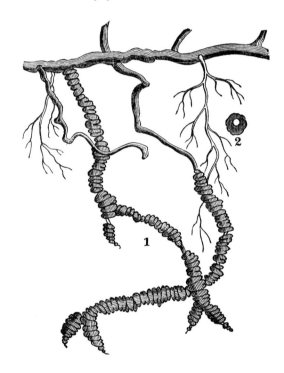

BLACK IPECACUANHA

Psychotria emetica

Class and Order, Pentandria Monogynia. Nat. Ord. Rubiaceæ.
Gen. Char. *Calix* five-toothed, coronated; *Corolla* tubular; *Berry* globose, seeds two, hemispherical, sulcated.— *Schreb.*

THIS genus, of which upwards of 90 species are enumerated, are principally confined to the warmer parts of the East and West Indies, growing in woods and shady places, particularly the herbaceous species. Numerous kinds possess emetic properties. The genus has been separated by recent authors and many of the species are distributed into other genera, or formed into new ones.

Psychotria emetica is more feeble in its effects, but similar in its operations with *Richardsonia emetica*; the roots are of a grayish black exteriorly, the woody part lighter coloured, but it is much greater in proportion than in the true drug, by which, as well as colour, it is readily distinguished from Cephaëlis or Richardsonia, and by its compact pith from the Ionidium. From its colour it is denominated Black Ipecacuanha.—G.

The various modes in which Ipecacuan acts on the system render it one of the most valuable articles of the Materia Medica.

In an uncombined form it acts, 1*st*, as an emetic; 2*dly*, as a tonic.

1. As an emetic, it is useful in all cases of poisoning where we wish to evacuate the stomach by causing vomiting; in poisoning with opium, it is preferable to all other emetics, as it neutralizes to a certain extent the narcotic influence of that substance, and as it has been known to succeed in evacuating the stomach, where sulphate of zinc and other more powerful emetics had previously failed. Dr Duncan says, "It (Ipecacuan) has frequently succeeded in stopping intermittent fevers, when given about an hour before an accession was expected, and also when given so as to produce vomiting at the time of an accession, or at the end of the cold stage." And again, "In continued fevers, we have never seen more decidedly beneficial effects from the use of any medicine whatever, than from the exhibition of ipecacuan in the primary stage of typhus fever. An emetic, succeeded by diluent diaphoretics, when administered sufficiently early in the disease, very frequently cuts it short; and when it fails in this desirable object, it always has a beneficial influence on the progress of the fever."

The common emetic dose, for an adult, is from a scruple to half a drachm, in a tea-cupful of hot water. Warm diluent drinks ought to be given, to promote the evacuation of the stomach.

2. As a tonic, Ipecacuan is often successful in restoring the healthy action of the stomach and intestines in dyspeptic habits, which have resisted the more common remedies of this class. One grain given twice or thrice a-day, and gradually increased to two or three grains, will be found to agree with most constitutions.

Combined with opium, Ipecacuan is known by the name of *Dover's powder*; it acts 1*st*, as a diaphoretic; 2*dly*, as an astringent.

1. *Dover's powder* is one of the best diaphoretics we possess; in rheumatism and in slight febrile affections, no remedy is more generally efficacious. Its dose, when given with the intention of causing diaphoresis, is from ten to twenty grains.

2. As an astringent, *Dover's* powder has been lately much employed for the cure of diarrhœa and dysentery. Even after the failure of *catechu, kino,* &c. chronic diarrhœas are often stopped by this medicine, and besides its astringent property, it seems to restore in a great measure the healthy secretion of the intestines. In Cholera spasmodica, *Dover's powder* has been given with the happiest effects, in doses of five or six grains, repeated three or four times in twenty-four hours.

Combined with squill and other expectorants, Ipecacuan, in doses of one or two grains, increases their power. Since the introduction and improved preparation of the *Muriate of Morphia* by Dr W. Gregory of Edinburgh, lozenges, composed of that substance in union with ipecacuan, have come into general use; and from the very good effects which have almost invariably resulted from their exhibition, they bid fair to cut out every other domestic pectoral remedy.

COMMON FENNEL

Fœniculum vulgare

Class and Order, PENTANDRIA DIGYNIA. NAT. ORD. UMBELLIFERÆ.
Gen. Char. *Calix* obsolete; *Petals* roundish, involute, narrower apex obtuse; *Fruit* nearly round; *Carpels* with five prominent obtuse-keeled ridges, of which the lateral ones are marginal and a little broader; *Interstices* with single vittæ, *Seed* subsemiterete; *Universal* and *partial involucres* wanting.

FENNEL is a common plant on various parts of Britain's coasts, particularly in chalky districts, and it is frequently met with amongst rubbish in the vicinity of towns; it has a tapering, fibrous, perennial root, which descends deep into the soil. Stems several, round, channelled, much branched, of a beautiful glaucous green, growing to the height of three or four feet; leaves much divided, the segments very slender; flowers of a full greenish-yellow. This species is very generally cultivated for culinary purposes, but the seeds, which are the official part, are usually imported from the south of Europe, and are known in the shops as Sweet Fennel seeds. The plant when cultivated acquires a milder taste and smell than it possesses in its wild state.

The seeds of the Fennel, like those of many other umbelliferous plants, are aromatic and carminative. They owe these virtues to the quantity of essential oil which they contain.

FOOLS PARSLEY

Æthusa cynapium

Class and Order, Pentandria Digynia. Nat. Ord. Umbelliferæ.
Gen. Char. *Calix* obsolete; *Petals* obcordate, with an inflexed point; *Fruit* ovato-globose; *Carpels* with five, elevated, thick, acutely carinated ridges, the lateral ones marginal and a little broader, bordered by a somewhat winged keel; *Interstices* with single *vittæ*; *Seed* semi-globose.—*Hooker.*

Root annual, stem one or two feet high, upright, branched, slightly grooved, hollow, covered with a bluish meal, which easily wipes off; leaves smooth, shining, of a deep green on the upper side, beneath paler and shining; sheaths of the foot-stalks small, smooth and membranous at their edges: the partial involucrum placed externally, and only surrounding one-half of the umbel, composed of three long, linear, pendulous leaves.

This species, which grows commonly in gardens and in waste places, has a considerable resemblance to the common parsley, likewise to the hemlock; from the former it is easily distinguished by its unpleasant odour; and from the latter, by its stems being without spots, and the three pendulous leaflets of its involucrum.

The *Æthusa cynapium* is a very active poison, and many fatal accidents have occurred from its having been eaten instead of parsley. Orfila mentions several cases of poisoning, among these,—one, of a child that ate a quantity of the leaves, and though it vomited them, became delirious, and supposed it saw dogs and cats; it was not seen by a medical man till next day, but it recovered. The same treatment which has been recommended under the head of *Œnanthe,* ought to be adopted.

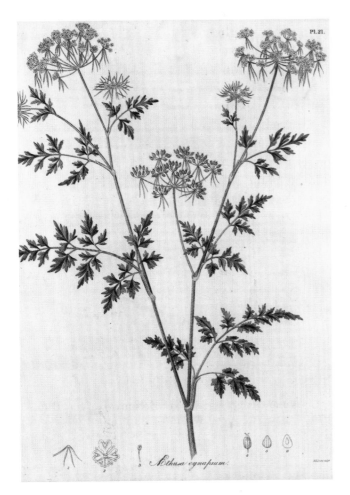

FOOLS PARSLEY

WILD CARROT

Daucus carota

Class and Order, Pentandria Digynia. Nat. Ord. Umbelliferæ.
Gen. Char. *Calix* of five teeth; *Petals* obcordate, point inflexed, the outer often radiant and deeply bifid; *Fruit* dorsally compressed; *Carpels* with five primary *ridges,* filiform and bristly, of which the three intermediate ones are dorsal, the two lateral ones on the inner face; the four *secondary ridges* equal, more prominent, with one row of prickles, which are slightly connected at the base; *Interstices* under the secondary ridges, with single *vittæ; Seed* plane in front; Universal and partial involucre many leaved, the former often primary.—*Hooker.*

The carrot in its wild state has a long tapering woody root; but by cultivation has been so altered, as to become the succulent root, so well known and esteemed for culinary and domestic purposes; it is found abundantly in pastures, borders of fields, and in hedge banks, and most abundantly on the sea coast. The whole plant is of closer growth, and much rougher in its wild state, than when under cultivation; the *D. maritima* is of a smaller size, with broader and more fleshy leaves, but both kinds vary so much, that they can hardly be considered as distinct species. Loudon enumerates fifteen species, besides three varieties of the cultivated kind, of which two only are natives of Britain.

Carrots abound in saccharine juice, and in France are used for the purpose of extracting their sugar. They are considered as by far the most nutritive of our esculent roots, for mankind as well as animals, and are by many considered as affording to horses and kine, equally substantial support as grain. A considerable variety are now cultivated, but generally those of a clear deep colour are more saccharine and better adapted for the table than the paler kinds.

The Seeds of the carrot are stimulant and diuretic, but are seldom prescribed. The roots when boiled and beaten to a pulp, form an excellent poultice for foul and cancerous sores; the pain and irritation are diminished, and the fœtor nearly destroyed during their application.

ANISE

Pimpinella anisum

Class and Order, PENTANDRIA DIGYNIA. NAT. ORD. UMBELLIFERÆ.
Gen. Char. *Calix* obsolete; *Petals* obcordate, with an inflexed point; *Fruit* laterally contracted, ovate, crowned with the swollen base of the reflected styles; *Carpels* with five filiform equal *ridges*, of which the lateral ones are marginal; *Interstices* with many *vittæ*; *Seed* gibbous, plane in front; *Universal* and *partial involucres* wanting.—*Hooker.*

ROOT annual, tapering; stem branched, smooth, striated, one foot to eighteen inches high; root leaves on longish channelled footstalks, of a somewhat roundish form, deeply divided into three or more lobes; cauline leaves becoming narrower upwards, divided into slender pinnated segments; flowers white, small, in terminal umbels.

Anise is a native of Egypt, but is cultivated in the southern parts of Europe; it is sufficiently hardy to bear temperate climates of Northern Europe but is not grown in sufficient quantity to supply the demand.

Anise-seeds are extensively used to flavour a spirituous cordial, known by the name of Aniseseed, and are possessed of a powerful scent, which has so fascinating a power on dogs that the oil is often employed for the purpose of decoying them away.

The volatile oil which is procured from the anise-seed by distillation is powerfully exciting, and in a large dose is capable of causing delirium. The carminative properties of this oil are of a very high order, and we find it much used along with oil of caraway in the colic of children. A celebrated empirical preparation, sold under the name of "Dalby's carminative," is supposed to owe its virtues to these oils united with water by means of magnesia. Expectorant properties are attributed to this oil.

HORSE-RADISH

Cochlearia armoracia

Class and Order, TETRADYNAMIA SILICULOSA. NAT. ORD. CRUCIFERÆ.
Gen. Char. *Pouch* oval or globose, many-seeded, valves ventricose; *Seeds* not margined; *Calix* spreading; *Petals* entire; *Stamens* without teeth.

A HARDY perennial of rapid growth, much disposed to become a troublesome weed in gardens, and cultivated grounds, though it is said to be found truly wild in some of the mountainous parts of England. It is of frequent occurrence amongst rubbish in uncultivated places, and as almost every part of the root will readily grow, it is easily established where any of the trimmings or cuttings of the root may be thrown. It is in much use as a condiment, and is largely cultivated for the table; its roots strike deep into the soil, and when once established, are by no means easy of extirpation.

The root of the horse-radish has an extremely pungent biting taste. An infusion is occasionally prescribed as a tonic in some scorbutic diseases, and in some varieties of dyspepsia, and very rarely in intermittents.

In Britain, horse-radish is chiefly cultivated as a culinary herb, but in France, it seems to be more esteemed as a medicine than as a condiment. Richard says that it is the most powerful, and the most active of antiscorbutics.

COMMON SWEET FLAG

Acorus calamus

Class and Order, HEXANDRIA MONOGYNIA. NAT. ORD. AROIDEÆ.
Gen. Char. *Flowers* arranged upon a spadix; *Spathe* wanting; *Perianth* of six pieces, scales inferior; *Stigma* sessile; *Capsule* indehiscent, many-seeded. *Hooker.*

Root perennial, extending horizontally, scarcely beneath the soil, throwing out numerous fibres which become thickly matted together; leaves long, undulated on one side, sword-shaped; flowers inconspicuous, growing upon a spadix from the leaf-like scape. There is no other indigenous plant with which this species can be confounded.

Acorus usually grows by the sides of rivers and in marshes, but it has succeeded very well with me when planted in a common border of the garden with a northern aspect. The root, which is the officinal part of the plant, is thick, internally white, externally yellowish green, of a spongy texture; it has an agreeable aromatic smell, and a warm pungent taste. The odour and taste are considerably increased by drying the root.

The root of the *Acorus calamus*, although seldom used either in this country or in France, is undoubtedly possessed of considerable power, as an aromatic and stimulant tonic; with this view, it is frequently used in Germany.

Dr Thomson recommends it as an addition to Cinchona and Quinine. He says that he has found these remedies, when combined with the *Acorus*, succeed in curing fevers which had resisted their effects when uncombined with it.

GARLIC

Allium sativum

Class and Order, Hexandria Monogynia. Nat. Ord. Liliaceæ.
Gen. Char. *Perianth* inferior, petaloid, of six ovate, spreading pieces; *Capsule* triquetrous.

Root perennial, formed of several bulbs enclosed in a common membrane; stem simple from one to two feet high; radical leaves numerous, long, plane, those on the stem few, and shorter than the others; flowers growing from a spathe, small, whitish green, intermixed with small bulbs: these latter, when the flowers are decayed, fall from the spathe and become new plants.

Garlic is a native of the southern parts of Europe, but is very generally cultivated for domestic and medicinal purposes. It increases rapidly by its roots, as well as being bulbiferous,

but the seed is very frequently abortive. Its odour is powerful, and to most persons excessively offensive; the scent is, with perhaps the exception of *A. ursinum*, the most unpleasant of all the tribe, the numerous species of which have in a greater or lesser degree the same smell.

Garlic is rarely prescribed internally in this country; it is occasionally employed as a stimulant cataplasm, but its disagreeable odour prevents its extensive use, as there are many equally efficacious rubefacients which are free of all unpleasant smell. A cataplasm of garlic applied to the pubes is said generally to succeed in procuring a discharge of urine, when the retention has arisen from want of due action of the bladder.

Garlic is used as a condiment, and enters into many of the epicure's sauces; in Spain, Portugal and Provence, the peasantry consume large quantities of it. The odour and rubefacient properties reside in an acrid essential oil, which is procured in the proportion of three-fourths of an ounce from twenty pounds of the root; it is so acrid, that when applied to the skin, it causes almost immediate vesication.

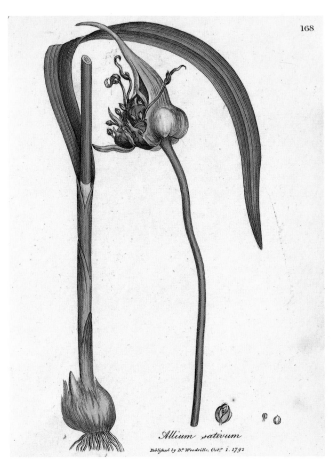

Allium sativum
Published by Dr Woodville, Oct.r 1. 1792

GARLIC

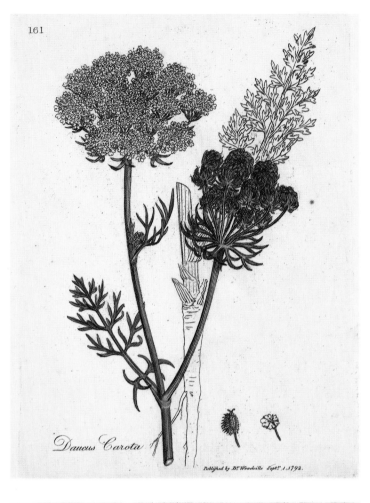

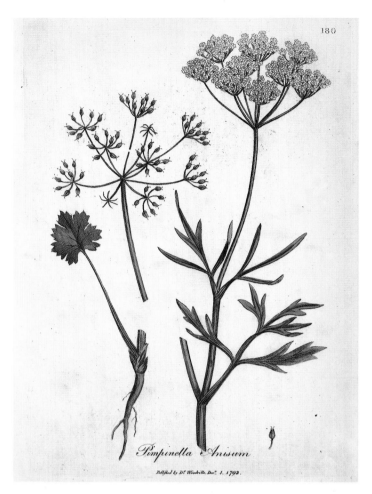

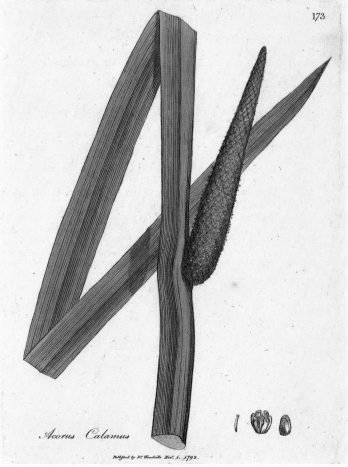

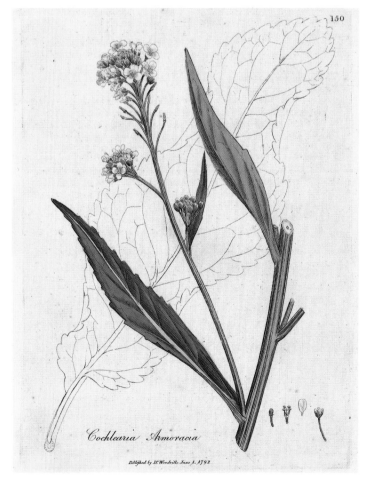

TOP LEFT: WILD CARROT, TOP RIGHT: ANISE, BOTTOM LEFT: COMMON SWEET FLAG,
BOTTOM RIGHT: HORSE-RADISH

ONION

Allium cepa

Class and Order, Nat. Ord. and Generic Character, see
A. sativum.

THE onion is too well known to require description. It possesses the properties of garlic in a milder form; is extensively used as an article of diet, and acts as a gentle stimulant. An essential oil is procured from it, possessing nearly the same properties as that of garlic.

COMMON LEEK

Allium porrum

Class and Order, Nat. Ord. and Generic Character, see
A. sativum.

THE Leek is a well known culinary vegetable, approaching the onion in taste and other properties, and is extensively cultivated for domestic purposes, particularly in the northern parts of Europe, being hardier than most of the cultivated Alliums. It is a native of Switzerland.

CALUMBO OR COLUMBO PLANT

Cocculus palmatus

Class and Order, DIŒCIA HEXANDRIA. NAT. ORD. MENIS-
PERMEÆ.
Gen. Char. *Sepals* and *Petals* in two series, rarely in three; *Stamens* six, free, opposite the petals; *Carpels* three to six; *Fruit* drupaceous, reniform, compressed, one-seeded; *Cotyledons* distant.—*De Candolle.*

ROOT perennial, thick, composed of a cluster of fleshy fusiform tubers growing from the parent root; stems annual, twining; leaves large, deeply divided into five or seven lobes; flowers growing in crowded spikes.

The plant producing the officinal columbo-root was long unknown in England, but is now satisfactorily ascertained to grow in thick forests that are said to cover the shores about Oibo and Mozambique, on the eastern coast of Africa, and inland for about fifteen or twenty miles, where it was long kept secret by the Portuguese, who alone traded in the drug. The male plant had been obtained in 1805, and was cultivated in the Mauritius, but the discovery of the female plant is more recent. Specimens with drawings of both sexes were transmitted by Mr Telfair to Dr Hooker, who published them in the Botanical Magazine, plates 2970 and 2971.

Calumbo root has been fraudulently imitated by slicing the roots of *Bryonia alba*, and when dry steeping them in a strong decoction of true Calumbo. The fictitious roots readily imbibe its colour and flavour, and that so completely, that specimens I prepared and gave to the late Dr A. Duncan could not be detected but by those well acquainted with the structure of the root. As will be observed in the annexed figures, besides the concentric circles, there are numerous radiating lines from the centre to the circumference, and whether the rings be numerous or only one, these lines are always present, and if the surface of the pieces under examination be cut smooth, the lines alone would detect the fallacy. In some specimens of the finest quality the lines are broken as in figure 2, or quite entire, extending from the bark to the centre, as in figures 1, and 3.

The colour of the dry pieces of the root are of a tolerably bright yellow, becoming paler towards the middle. In one of Dr Hooker's figures the whole of the inner part of the root is represented of a full yellow. This is not the case in a root I have before me, where the depth of colour is confined to the first ring next the bark, gradually fading to almost white, but is dark or brownish in the centre. Some years ago, the demand for this drug induced numerous frauds; but the great reduction in its value, renders it now not worth the trouble of imitating.

The finest samples of the drug are of a bright yellow colour, becoming paler towards the middle, which is usually clouded. It should break short, and have a full but not unpleasant bitter taste, and be quite free from worm holes.

Calumbo belongs to the class of simple bitters. It is one of the most valuable we possess, and is much more grateful than most of its class. It is useful in dyspepsia arising from want of tone in the digestive organs, in chronic diarrhœas, and in cholera. In the last mentioned disease it ought to be combined with opium or morphia. In diarrhœa, the addition of a small quantity of chalk and rhubarb is advisable. Richard says, that it is but reasonable to attribute part of its efficacy in diarrhœa, dysentery, and obstinate vomiting, to the starch which it contains.

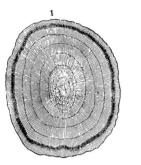
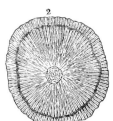
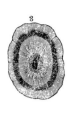

WHITE OR RED BERRIED BRYONY

Bryonia dioica

Class and Order, Monoecia Polyandria. Nat. Ord. Cucurbitaceæ.
Gen. Char. Male flower; *Calix* five-toothed; *Corolla* five cleft; *Filaments* three; *Anthers* five.
Female flower; *Calix* five toothed; *Corolla* five cleft; *Style* trifid; *Berry* inferior, globose, many-seeded.

In England, particularly in the southern parts, the Bryony is exceedingly common, being to be met with in almost every hedge-row; but in other parts of the kingdom it is comparatively scarce, and it can hardly be considered as a native of Scotland.

Root very large, from eight inches to a foot or more in diameter, of an irregular form, with fibres sparingly produced on all sides, penetrating deep into the soil, and tapering towards the extremity; stems numerous, long, weak, straggling, and frequently taking nearly a horizontal direction under ground, furnished with tendrils, and generally climbing; leaves large, palmate, and, as well as most other parts of the plant, sparingly furnished with thick glandulous hairs; flowers growing in clusters, the male and female flowers on different plants; berries at first green, but becoming a bright red when ripe. This plant is in common use as a laxative among the gardeners and labouring men in the south of England, who prepare the root by first cleansing it of all extraneous substances, then cutting it into small pieces, and steeping these in spirit (common gin;) after two or three days it is fit for use. The usual practice, is to fill a wine bottle as nearly as possible with the pieces of the fresh root, and add as much spirit as will cover it. The root if good will bear spirit to be added to it several times. It is more acrid when in full flower and before the berries begin to change colour;

but the root contains a greater quantity of juice during the winter season, though its taste at this time is less nauseous. The common dose is a small tea-cup full.

It is of very quick growth, and in a congenial soil will extend its stalks many yards round, provided it meets with anything around which its tendrils can entwine for support; but if suffered to trail on the ground, its growth is much stunted; its leaves are very subject to be devoured by caterpillars, and I have several times met with the *Sphinx ligustri*, the privet hawk-moth, hovering over the flower, many evenings in succession.

The root of the Bryony has an extremely nauseous bitter taste, and acts as a violent purgative. It is not now used in medicine. When given in a moderate dose, it causes copious watery evacuations, accompanied with nausea, vomiting, and tormina; in a large dose, it acts as an acrid poison, causing death in a very short time. Orfila mentions a case where death took place in four hours, from the decoction of half an ounce of the root.

COMMON SORREL

Rumex acetosa

Class and Order, Hexandria Trigynia. Nat. Ord. Polygoneæ.
Gen. Char. *Calix* of three leaves, united at the base; *Corolla* of three petals; *Stigmas* multifid; *Nut* triquetrous, covered by the enlarged petals, which often bear tubercles.—*Hooker*.

Sorrel is a common plant, growing abundantly in fields and meadows throughout the kingdom. Its root is perennial, stalk upright, channelled, branched at the top, one or two feet high, radical leaves arrow-shaped on long footstalks, the cauline sessile, and alternate; flowers at the extremity of the branches of a green colour, with red or purplish veins. This plant, as well as the *acetosella* and *scutatis*, are often eaten as salad; the latter species is grown on the continent for that purpose; this section of the *Rumices* contain only plants that abound in an agreeable acid.

It is to the bin-oxalate of potass, which the leaves of the *Rumex acetosa* contain, that they owe their cooling properties; an infusion of the leaves forms a very agreeable drink in fevers and inflammatory diseases. A very curious, and at the same time important property, is attributed to the juice of this plant; it is that of destroying the acrimony of acrid vegetables, both before and after they have been swallowed. If the leaves of the Rumex be bruised along with those of one of the Ranunculaceæ, the latter lose their acrimony. The leaves of the *Arum* are also said to become mild and innoxious when treated in the same way. This subject deserves the utmost attention.

COMMON BROOM

Cytisus scoparius

Class and Order, Diadelphia Decandria. Nat. Ord. Leguminosæ.
Gen. Char. *Calix* two lipped, the upper lip nearly entire, or with two small teeth, lower one three-toothed; *Standard* large, broadly ovate; *Keel* very blunt, including the stamens; *Legume* flattened, many-seeded.

The Broom is abundant on commons, heaths, and barren places; it forms a shrub from three to six feet high, very much branched, the branches upright, twiggy, green, angular, flexible, the young ones downy. It produces a profusion of flowers early in the spring, and merits a place in every extensive plantation or garden. It varies with double flowers, and sometimes its blossoms are of a deep orange colour.

The leaves, young shoots, and seeds of the broom are diuretic, and in large doses emetic and purgative. A decoction of the young shoots is a favourite popular remedy in gravel and dysuria. In the seeds I found a substance analogous to the *Cytisine* obtained from the *Cytisus laburnum* and *Arnica montana*, and procured by a somewhat similar process, which, as well as its effects on animals, will be described under the head of *Arnica montana*.

BURDOCK

Arctium lappa

Class and Order, Syngenesia Æqualis. Nat. Ord. Cichoraceæ , Tribe II. Cinarocephaleæ.
Gen. Char. *Involucre* globose, each of its scales with an incurved hook at the extremity; *Receptacle* chaffy; *Pappus* simple.

A common plant, to be met with in waste places, road sides, and more seldom in fields. Its lower leaves attain to a large size; its stalks in the young state are often used for culinary purposes, and the roots are sometimes boiled and brought to table, for which purpose both root and stalks should be procured before the flowers expand, otherwise they become woody. There are two varieties of this plant, which have been considered as distinct species; the common one figured on the annexed plate and the *Bardana*; the heads of the latter are often thickly coated with a fine cottony substance resembling spider's web, but as they are to be met with in all stages between the perfectly free and densely coated heads, they can with propriety be only considered as varieties of the same species.

The heads or burrs, are, from their construction, admirably adapted for dispersion, by the hooked scales of the receptacle adhering to the skins and furs of animals, and the species is abundant over the whole of Britain.

A decoction of the roots of the burdock is occasionally prescribed as a diaphoretic, and is highly spoken of by some authors, among others by Richard. The late Dr Duncan employed it occasionally as a substitute for Sarsparilla with very good effect. In various parts of the Conti-

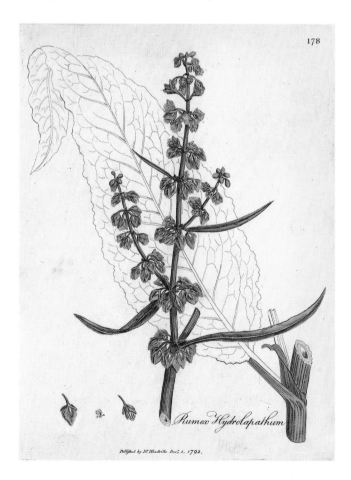

Rumex Hydrolapathum

Published by W. Woodville Decr 1, 1792.

COMMON SORREL

nent the roots are eaten by the peasantry, and are said to resemble artichokes. While analyzing the roots of the *Arctium*, I found a peculiar colouring matter which possesses the power of changing colour in a very remarkable manner. When the decoction is filtered, it is of a pale yellow; on the addition of ammonia the yellow deepens to orange, and if the liquid be immediately corked up, it will continue of that colour for years. When, however, it is exposed to the air for a few hours, it gradually assumes a greenish tinge, and at the expiration of eight or ten hours, every vestige of the yellow will have disappeared, and the liquid will have become of a green, more or less intense according to the strength of the decoction. After this change, if the green liquid be again put into a vessel closely stopped, yellow will again appear in a few days, and at the end of a fortnight or so, the orange will be completely restored. I have some portions of a decoction made four years since, which still exhibit this property of changing colour. To ensure its keeping for so long a time, it is necessary to add about a fifth part of alcohol.

ANGUSTURA BARK

Galipea officinalis

Class and Order, Diandria Monogynia. Nat. Ord. Rutaceæ.
Gen. Char. *Calix* short, five-toothed; *Corolla* somewhat campanulate, deeply cut into five segments; *Stamens* four, two of which are sterile.

The plant producing the true Angustura Bark, has been arranged in various genera by different authors. I had adopted the name of Bonplandia, as given by Humboldt, which is the one engraved on the accompanying plate; but, finding Aublet's provincial name of Galipea recognized by most modern authors on the ground of priority, I have retained it.

This tree grows to sixty or eighty feet high, and is a native of South America, where it was first clearly ascertained by the celebrated Humboldt, and is accurately figured in his *Plantes Equinoxiales*. The true Angustura Bark is readily known from the spurious by the colour as well as texture. I have figured both on the annexed plate, which will supersede the necessity of further description.

Angustura bark was introduced into Euro-

pean practice about forty years since; it is highly extolled by the Americans as a remedy in intermittent fevers, and in dysentery: it has also been recommended in yellow fever. When any inflammatory symptoms are present, its employment is contraindicated, as it is a highly stimulating tonic.

ANTIDYSENTERIC BRUCEA OR FALSE ANGUSTURA BARK

Brucea antidysenterica

Class and Order, Dioecia Tetrandria. Nat. Ord. Rutaceæ.
Gen. Char. Flowers of separate sexes; *Calix* four parted; *Petals* four, hardly equal the length of the calix.
Male Flower; *Stamens* four, short inserted round about a gland-like central four-lobed body.
Female Flower; *Stamens* four, sterile; *Ovaries* four, seated on a four-lobed receptacle, each terminated by a simple acute reflexed stigma; *Drupes* four, one-seeded.—*Don.*

This species is described by Don as a shrub of eight feet high. For the specimens from which the accompanying figures were taken, I am indebted to the kindness of Dr Christison; and I have contrasted them on the same plate with that of the true Angustura Bark, the more clearly to show the difference of structure in the two kinds; the epidermis in the *Bonplandia* is thin, and adheres closely to the liber; that of the Brucea is thick, and much resembles in appearance a crustaceous Lichen; its taste is intensely bitter, and it leaves a burning sensation in the throat, which continues for many hours. I chewed and swallowed a small piece, not exceeding in size half a hemp-seed, and for the greater part of that day I suffered exceedingly from dryness of the throat, which lasted for at least eight hours. In the smaller piece, Fig. 3, the inner side of the bark was pale-coloured, as in the figure, but in all other respects resembled the others, and possessed the same properties.

The unpleasant effects which have been attributed to Angustura Bark, are now traced to the *Brucea antidysenterica*, which is occasionally met with under the name of Angustura, and has acquired the name of "False Angustura Bark." The accidents which occurred from the substitution of this for the true bark were at one time so numerous as to induce the Austrian and some other governments, to interdict the importation

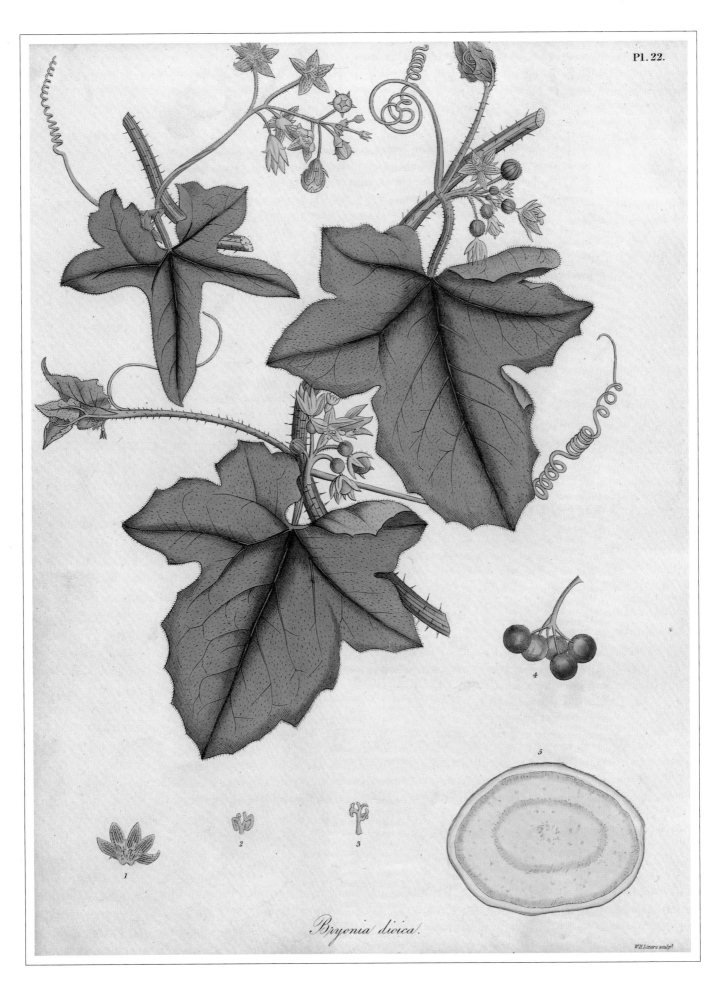

Pl. 22.

Bryonia dioica.

W.H.Lizars sculpt.

WHITE OR RED BERRIED BRYONY; FIG.1, A FLOWER LAID OPEN; FIG.2, STAMENS;
FIG.3, PISTILS; FIG.4, FRUIT; FIG.5, TRANSVERSE SECTION OF THE ROOT.

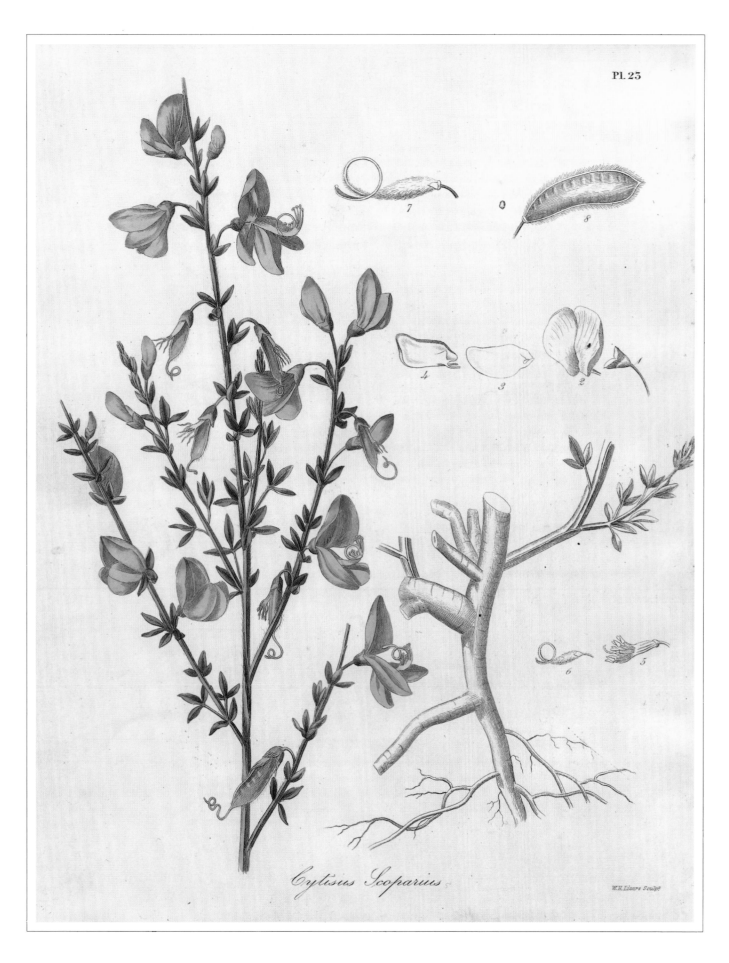

Pl. 23

Cytisus Scoparius.

W.H. Lizars Sculp.

COMMON BROOM; FIG.1, CALIX; FIG.2, VEXILLUM; FIG.3, ALOEA; FIG.4, CARINA;
FIG.5, STAMENS; FIG.6, PISTIL; FIG.7, SEED-VESSEL IN A YOUNG STATE; FIG.8,
LEGUME; FIG.9, SEED.

of the Angustura itself, and to order the destruction of all that already imported. Pelletier and Caventou ascertained by analysis, that the Brucea owes its poisonous qualities to the presence of an alkaloid, to which they have given the name of *Brucia*, or *Brucine*; it exists in the form of a gallate, and in considerable quantity, as though the alkaloid is only one-twelfth, or, according to some, one twenty-fourth part as strong as Strychnia, yet eight grains of the bark proved fatal to a dog, which shows it to be nearly as powerful a poison as the Nux vomica itself. The symptoms produced are nearly the same as those caused by Nux vomica, viz. violent convulsions, succeeded by tetanus.

In cases of poisoning from the Brucea, ether and other stimuli ought to be freely administered. Dr Christison remarks, that during the intervals which occur between the spasmodic paroxysms the intellect is very acute.

PERUVIAN OR JESUITS' BARK

Cinchona

Class and Order, PENTANDRIA MONOGYNIA. NAT. ORD. RUBIACEÆ.
Gen. Char. *Corolla* monopetalous, funnel-shaped; *Capsule* inferior, two celled; *Seeds* numerous, oblong, compressed, winged.

THE drugs known in commerce and medicine by the name of Peruvian bark or Cinchona, are obtained from South America, but other species are dispersed through the East and West Indies, the Philippine, and South Sea Islands. The Peruvian Bark is now held of the utmost importance in every part of the known world where the healing art is scientifically practised, yet up to the present period we are in uncertainty as to the species producing the various kinds in common use.

Two centuries have passed away since this drug was first introduced into European practice, and though for a great length of time it shared the fate that all new medicines, however valuable, have encountered from the hostility of interested or ignorant practitioners, its virtues were of that intrinsic kind that survive the prejudice of the times. When its real value was duly appreciated, the drug became a monopoly in the hands of the Jesuits, from whence it derived one of its older names, Jesuits' bark. At

that period, in the priest were commonly combined the professions of medicine and theology; and we find that in most countries where the Roman Catholic is the established region, the same practice obtains in some degree to the present day.

The officinal Cinchonas are natives of the mountainous forests of Peru, extending from the fourth degree of north latitude, and growing on mountains of from 3000 to 9000 feet in altitude. A. B. Lambert, Esq. has enumerated in his illustration of the genus, twenty-two species, and forty-four kinds of bark; but it is not a little remarkable, that with this considerable acquaintance with the family, the identical species which produce the principal barks of commerce are by no means satisfactorily ascertained.

The Cinchonas form trees from thirty to one hundred feet high, but from the destruction constantly going forward in the Cinchona forests, they are rarely found of any considerable magnitude at the present day; few specimens of the bark reach this country that appear to belong to any but either very small trees or branches. It is highly probable that other species exist of equal value to those I have enumerated, but the quantity of active principles contained in the barks, *quinine* and *cinchonine*, differ greatly in the different kinds. Some specimens I examined under the name of Potoya Bark, were equal in flavour to the best Crown bark; that known as the Carthagena bark, is often met with, but is in little estimation. The Silver bark is likewise of but little value, though in some countries it is thought to possess considerable virtues.

YELLOW BARK

Cinchona cordifolia

Cinchona *cordifolia*; leaves heart-shaped at the base, roundish ovate, acute; panicle branched, pubescent; calix five-toothed, the segments broad, rounded, terminated by a mucro; capsule smooth, ovate-oblong.

THE Yellow Bark is of recent introduction into European practice, and was brought to England about the year 1790; it is of a deeper colour than the pale bark, and bears a great resemblance to that kind. It is usually imported in larger pieces than the Pale or Crown Bark; it is of a more powerfully bitter taste; and is commonly met with in flat pieces, as represented at figure 5. Its appearance is fibrous, but it breaks short with a shining fracture. The flat yellow bark is generally without its epidermis, and is often mixed with splints of the wood; the quilled kind usually loses its epidermis, and is in every direction traversed by deep fissures. Its surface, on removing the epidermis (in the larger pieces) is dark-brown, but beneath is of the same bright orange-yellow as the inner side. The smaller pieces of quilled bark seem to have their epidermis destroyed by the numerous lichens with which it abounds; these are generally of a grey, almost white colour. The small quills are commonly paler coloured than the flat or larger quilled kind, and are figured in several varieties, at 1, 2, 3, 4. It may be proper to notice, that those pieces which on examination have their pores filled by a shining resinous matter, are accounted of less value than those in which the texture of the bark is visible without the resin.

The Yellow Bark, which is the one most commonly prescribed, is a powerful febrifuge and tonic. When powdered, it ought to be of a bright-yellow, with a slight tinge of orange.

PALE OR CROWN BARK

Cinchona condaminea

Cinchona *condaminea*; leaves ovate lanceolate, smooth, shining, beneath having little hollows at the axils of the veins; panicle much branched; teeth of the calix ovate acuminate; corolla silky, segments ovate acuminate; capsule oblong.

THIS species is supposed to produce the pale or crown bark of the shops, but as several figures of the plant are published which are copied from each other, I consider it unnecessary to add another. On the annexed Plate, are represented at figs. 1, 2, 3, specimens of the finest pale quilled bark; which has a pale-greyish or ash-coloured epidermis, frequently blotched with various species of lichen and parasitic fungi. In substance it is about the eighth of an inch thick, mostly quilled; the inner surface of a pale cinnamon colour, of a resinous appearance, breaking short, and is friable between the teeth; its taste is bitter, but with somewhat of an aromatic flavour, and it is one of the pleasantest of the *Cinchonæ*. Mixed with this is often found

a thinner sort of a duller colour, with the epidermis of an uniform dull-brown, and having the inner side much duller than the previous kind; it differs also in having the circular fissures in the epidermis nearly obsolete, whilst in the finer kinds, these rings are deep and broad, and often appear as if occasioned by ligatures having been tightly fastened: it is represented at fig. 6, and is much inferior to either the pale or crown bark; is much thinner, more fibrous, and has less taste, and this, frequently with a slight admixture of mustiness. It commonly has the same parastical fungi and lichens. Crown Bark, which is esteemed as a variety obtained from the same species as the two foregoing, is held in great repute, and acquired its appellation from its being reserved for the exclusive use of the royal household of Spain. It is of a much darker colour on the exterior, but internally resembles the pale bark in its fracture and taste, but the latter is more intensely bitter. The lichens found on this kind, differ from those on the foregoing; besides various small patches of uncertain figure which are distributed on the surface, a light bluish-grey pulverulent kind is scattered in blotches, that give it an ash-coloured appearance. It is represented at figures 4 and 5.

The Pale, Grey, or Crown Bark, is the mildest and least nauseous of the genus, and is more frequently prescribed as a tonic than as a febrifuge. It derives the name of Pale from the colour of its powder, which is of a much lighter shade than that of either the Yellow or Red Bark. The name of Grey Bark is derived from the colour of its epidermis.

RED BARK

Cinchona oblongifolia

Cinchona *oblongifolia*; leaves oblong, broad, ovate, smooth, and shining, beneath tomentose; panicles corymbose, branched, woolly; corolla with spreading lanceolate segments, hairy within; capsule ovate.

THE substance of Red Bark is coarse and heavy, of a deep but dull red colour on the outside; within brighter. It is fibrous, but breaks short, and is friable between the teeth; it is usually imported in flat pieces without the epidermis, as at figure 6, but is occasionally met with quilled; the epidermis of the smaller pieces is of a dull greyish-brown, and it is generally invested with numerous lichens, mostly of a white or cream-colour; these, as at fig. 4, seem to absorb or destroy the epidermis. I have some specimens which are so close and heavy as to sink in water. From the discordant opinions of botanists, it is pretty certain that the tree producing the red bark is not ascertained.

The most powerful, and at the same time the most disagreeable of the cinchonæ, is the Red Bark; it never was so highly esteemed as either of the foregoing, but from the quantity of the active principles which it contains, it may be regarded as among the most valuable species in commerce.

The natural family of the Rubiaceæ (Cinchonaceæ of Lindley), produces many medicinal plants of very great value, among which *Cinchona* and *Cephaelis* are pre-eminent. The genus Cinchona includes a great variety of species, differing a good deal from each other in strength, but all possessing, as far as we are acqainted with them, febrifuge or tonic virtues. The mode in which the febrifuge properties of this genus became first known is uncertain: the discovery is usually attributed to the Jesuits; but whether they derive their information from the Peruvians, or whether they made the discovery themselves, is not ascertained. The name *Cinchona* is said to have been given to this drug, from the circumstance of a Countess of Cinchona, the wife of the Viceroy of Lima, having been cured of fever by the use of it. Although many eminent physicians opposed the use of cinchona on its first introduction, and for some time afterwards, we find its virtues have been pretty generally acknowledged and appreciated, since the middle of the 17th century.

As a febrifuge, it is prescribed in intermittent and remittent fevers, and also in continued fever; in the latter, however, it ought only to be employed in the debility which follows the disease, or when typhoid symptoms present themselves; in the first stage, or that of excitement, the use of so stimulating a substance would be injurious; in intermittent fevers, considerable difference of opinion exists with regard to the period at which the dose ought to be given, some advocating the administration immediately before the accession, others immediately after it, and others during the whole intervals between the fits. Richard recommends it to be given seven or eight hours before the accession, in which case, he says, the medicine has time to operate before the hour at which the accession takes place. He reprobates the idea of giving it immediately before or during the accession, as in this case the violence of the fit is increased. In remittent fever, the same author advises that the bark should be administered towards the end of one exacerbation, so as to moderate or prevent the next.

In all diseases in which there is a tendency to gangrene or putrescency, cinchona is one of the most valuable remedies we possess. In hospital gangrene, in confluent small-pox, putrid sore throat, and erysipelatous inflammation, large and repeated doses, combined with diffusible stimuli and the mineral acids, are frequently successful. As a tonic, cinchona is useful in all cases in which there is constitutional debility, uncombined with organic disease, in dyspepsia arising from loss of tone, in diarrhœas which have lasted for a length of time, in contagious dysentery, in scurvy, in passive hemorrhage, and in some varieties of hæmoptysis. Dr Haygarth has mentioned the efficacy of cinchona in curing rheumatism even without the assistance of venesection or any of the usual means employed for the cure of that disease. In dropsy, as a general tonic, it sometimes succeeds in preventing a return after the water has been evacuated either by medicine or by tapping. In malignant ulcers in which the edges are flabby, and where there is an obvious want of proper action, cinchona may be advantageously prescribed both as an internal remedy, and as an external application.

Though the discovery of the active principles of Cinchona, has rendered the exhibition of the bark or its preparations of rarer occurrence than formerly, yet as some practitioners prefer it, and as in some instances it may be more efficacious or convenient, it may be as well to mention shortly what are considered the best modes of giving it. The powder, which is by many considered the best preparation, is to many persons extremely nauseous and cannot be persevered in from the sickness to which it gives rise,—the addition of half a grain of opium (when it is admissible), or of half a drachm of some aromatic powder, such as cinnamon, will in most cases prevent this disagreeable effect, but if not, recourse must be had to the infusion or tincture,

Pl. 24.

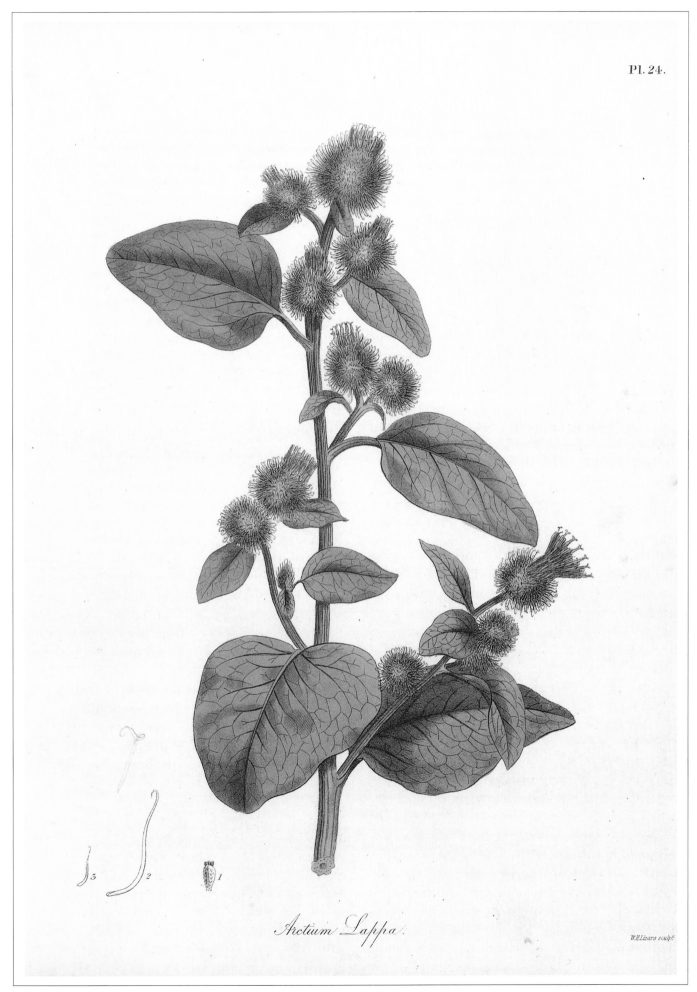

Arctium Lappa.

W.H.Lizars sculp.t

BURDOCK

which are less apt to occasion unpleasant effects.

Quinine and *cinchonine* possess all the tonic and febrifuge virtues of the Cinchonæ in a concentrated form, but their insolubility renders them ineligible as remedies. They are always prescribed, united with an acid, and of the salts formed the sulphates are the most generally used. Of these the sulphate of *quinine* is by far the most commonly prescribed. In general debility, in the dyspepsia of weak habits, and in intermittent and remittent fevers, it is a sovereign remedy. In all diseases which return periodically, in rheumatism, in tic douloureux, it has succeeded after the failure of the more ordinary modes of treatment.

As a tonic, the sulphate of *quinine* is given in doses of from one to two grains, twice or thrice a day, either in the form of pill or in solution.

As a febrifuge, the dose varies with the character of the fever. It is usual to begin with two or three grains twice a-day, and gradually to increase the dose to seven or eight, or even more. The increase must be regulated by the effects. In rheumatism the quantity given is much larger. Dr Duncan, who was among the first to use it, gave ten or twelve grains twice or thrice a-day, and in one case, I recollect of its having been administered in scruple doses with the most complete success.

In tic douloureux, the dose ought also to be large. If the constitution suffer much disturbance, the dose must of course be lessened, and the remedy intermitted if necessary.

COMMON CUCKOO-FLOWER OR LADY'S SMOCK

Cardamine pratensis

Class and Order, Tetradynamia Siliquosa. Nat. Ord. Cruciferæ.
Gen. Char. *Pod* linear, the valves flat, generally separating elastically, nerveless, seedstalks slender; *Cotyledons* accumbent.

This is a most abundant species, being found in profusion in almost every moist pasture or wet meadow throughout Britain, producing its lively purple (sometimes white) flowers, towards the end of April or beginning of May; it has acquired the common name of Cuckoo-flower, from the circumstance of its blossoms expanding about the time the Cuckoo visits this country; it is frequently found with double flowers both wild and cultivated, and this variety increases rapidly by its leaves, all of which growing in contact with the ground, throw out fibres from both the upper and under sides, and when once rooted the footstalk of the leaf decays.

At one time the *Cardamine pratensis* was in some repute as a diuretic; it is now never used in medicine, but is occasionally eaten instead of the water-cress, which it resembles in taste. Diaphoretic properties are attributed to it.

SAVINE

Juniperus sabina

Class and Order, Nat. Ord. and Generic Character, see
J. communis.
Juniperus *sabina*; leaves opposite, blunt, glandular in the middle, imbricated in four ways; stem shrubby.

The Savine is of very similar form and mode of growth to the common juniper, but its berries are smaller, and closely surround the stalks; it is a native of the south of Europe, but grows readily in Britain, when it will form a low, close, evergreen bush, three or four feet high. We learn from Turner's Herbal that it was cultivated in Britain so long ago as the year 1562.

The leaves of the *Juniperus sabina* have a disagreeable, bitter, and somewhat acrid taste, and yield by distillation an essential oil, possessing all their qualities in a concentrated degree. Savine is diaphoretic, stimulant, and emmenagogue. In a large dose it is said to cause abortion; and as it is frequently resorted to for that purpose, it becomes an object of interest to medical jurists. Dr Christison, treating of the subject, says: "Doubts, however, may be entertained, whether any such property is possessed by it, independently of its action as a violent acrid on the bowels. It has certainly been taken to a considerable extent, without the intended effect; of which Foderé has noticed an unequivocal example. A woman took daily, for twenty days, no less than an hundred drops of the oil, yet carried her child to the full term. The powder has likewise been taken to a large extent without avail. The same author remarks, that, if given in sufficient quantity to cause violent purging, abortion may ensue, but, unless in those cases in which there is a predisposition to miscarriage,

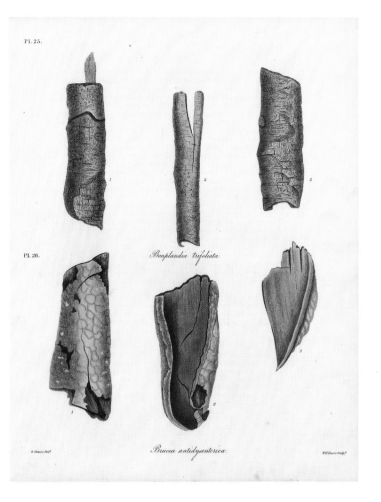

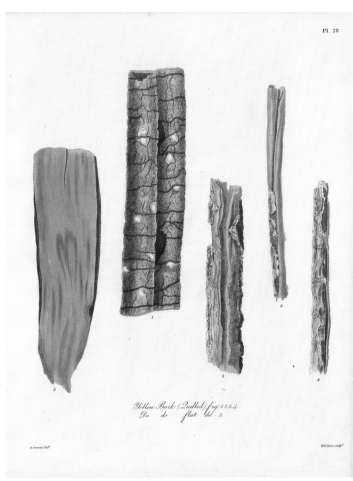

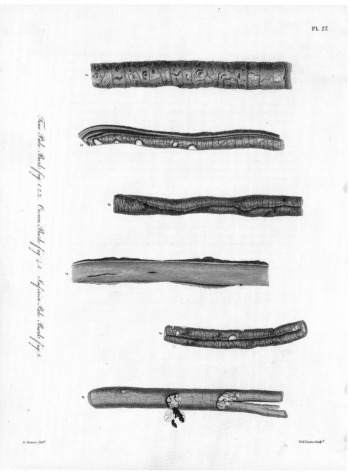

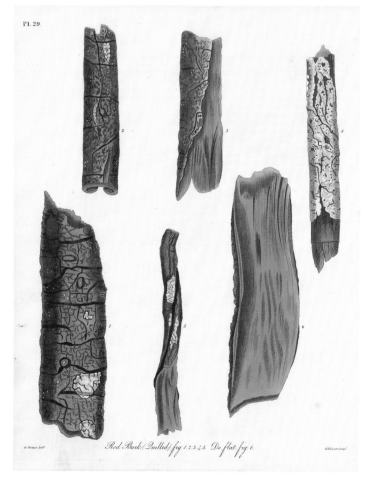

TOP LEFT: ANGUSTURA BARK AND ANTIDYSENTERIC BRUCEA, TOP RIGHT: YELLOW
BARK, BOTTOM LEFT: JESUIT'S BARK AND CROWN BARK, BOTTOM RIGHT: RED BARK

the constitutional injury and intestinal irritation required to induce it are so great, as to be always attended with great danger, independent of the uterine disorder." Again, "in a charge of wilful abortion, the mere possession of oil of savine would be a suspicious circumstance, because the notion that it has the power of causing miscarriage is very general and familiar with the vulgar, while it is scarcely employed for any useful purpose. The leaves in the form of infusion, are in some parts of England a popular remedy for worms." Orfila has given the result of his experiments on dogs, from which it is obviously one of the class of acrid poisons. An ointment made by boiling the leaves in lard, is a good deal used for keeping up a discharge from blistered surfaces, and for stimulating old sores.

COMMON WOOD SORREL

Oxalis acetosella

Class and Order, Decandria Pentagynia. Nat. Ord. Oxalideæ.

Gen. Char. *Calix* five-parted; *Petals* five, free or sometimes united together at the base; *Stamens* ten, filaments frequently connected at the base, the five outer ones shorter than the others; *Capsule* angular, five-celled; *Cells* two or many-seeded; *Seeds* with an elastic arillus.

Root perennial, horizontal, scaly, with a few straggling fibres; leaves on long, slender, reddish footstalks. The leaflets fold together and droop at night, and during wet weather. Flowers large, usually white, elegantly striped with purple veins; seed-vessel bursting on being slightly handled; and towards the end of summer, it frequently produces perfect capsules and seeds, without any appearance of corolla; as is common with several species of *Violet*.

It is subject to considerable variety in the colour of its flowers. In some the blossoms are a pale bluish tint, and it is then the var. β. of Decandolle; in others they are pale rose coloured, when it is var. γ. of the same author. The genus is very extensive; two hundred and twenty-three species are described in Don's System of Gardening, only two of which are natives of Britain.

Wood sorrel is found in shady woods and coppices, also among stones and rocks at a great elevation, on some of the highest mountains in Scotland. It is a plant of easy cultivation, and from its beauty is well worth the attention of the horticulturist.

The Wood sorrel contains a considerable portion of the bin-oxalate of potass, which communicates to its juice the pleasant acid for which it is so well known. An infusion made from the leaves forms a pleasant cooling drink. At one period, the bin-oxalate of potass, which is well known by the name of "Essential salt of Lemons," was prepared entirely from this plant, and from the *Rumex acetosa*.

While prepared in this manner, the salt was expensive, as only about a drachm was obtained from a pound of the fresh plant. In 1827, Scheele published a process for preparing this salt, by the addition of potass to oxalic acid, and in this way, all the bin-oxalate used in medicine, or for domestic purposes, is prepared. A weak solution, sweetened with sugar, is sometimes given as a cooling drink in fevers and inflammatory diseases.

Oxalic acid is more frequently used for the purpose of removing stains, than this salt, as it acts much more readily, and with greater certainty.

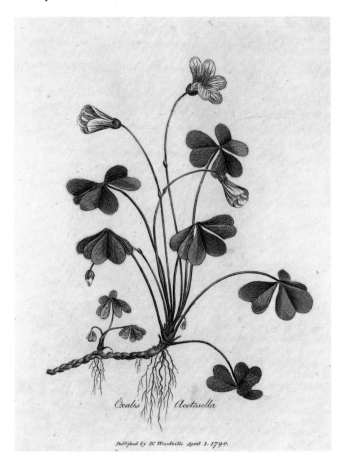

Oxalis Acetosella

Published by Dr. Woodville April 1. 1790.

COMMON WOOD SORREL

A short time since a paper appeared in the Journal of the Royal Institution, in which the author proves, or attempts to prove, that the *Oxalis acetosella* is the true shamrock.

COMMON JUNIPER

Juniperus communis

Class and Order, Diœcia Monadelphia. Nat. Ord. Coniferæ.
Gen. Char. Male Flowers; *Scales* of the *Catkin* subpeltate; *Perianth* wanting; *Stamens* four to eight, one-celled. Female Flowers; *Scales* of the *Catkin* few, united, at length fleshy, and surrounding the three-seeded *berry*.

A HARDY perennial shrub, varying in size according to the situation and altitude in which it grows, at times reaching several feet in height, and at others being almost prostrate. Its branches are much divided, and thickly beset with numerous long, pointed, dark-green leaves. It flowers in May, and its berries continue on the bush for two years before they are ripe, when

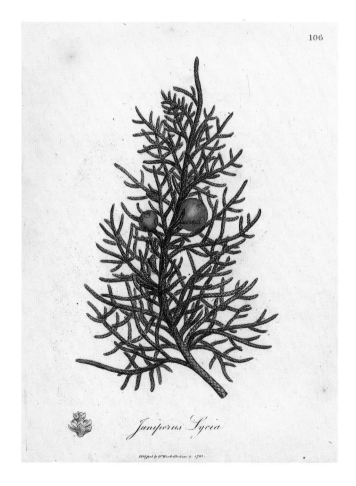

Juniperus Lycia

Published by Wm Woodville June 1. 1793.

COMMON JUNIPER

they are of a bluish-black colour. They are much used to flavour spirits, and communicate the peculiar flavour so much admired in Hollands.

This species is dispersed over all the northern parts of Europe and America, and is abundantly met with on dry elevated places. In the procumbent state of the plant it has been described by some authors as a distinct species, under the name of *J. nana*, but as above stated it may be found in all varieties of form, from a low trailing shrub to a bush several feet high. In Loudon's Hortus Britannicus twenty-four species are enumerated.

The berries of the Juniper have a sweetish, somewhat aromatic, taste; they are stimulant carminative, tonic, and diuretic.

The essential oil has the peculiar flavour of the berries, and possesses their diuretic and stimulating properties. To its presence Hollands owes its peculiar flavour; English gin ought also to be prepared from it, but in the preparation of this spirit, oil of turpentine is used in large quantities, often without the smallest admixture of oil of juniper. The Dutch, in making Hollands, do not first distil the oil and then add it to the spirit; they submit the berries to the process of fermentation along with the malt, and then proceed with the distillation. Both the decoction and extract are mere weak bitters, the greater part of the oil being dissipated in their preparation.

CATHARTIC CROTON

Croton tiglium

Class and Order, Nat. Ord. and Generic Character, see
C. Eleutheria.

THE plant which produces the seeds from which the croton oil is expressed is a native of various parts of India and the adjacent islands. It grows to the height of fifteen to twenty feet, forming a low handsome tree with extending branches; the bark is blackish, covered with small gray lichens.

Persoon has enumerated eighty-two species, but other botanists have removed many of them into other genera; the *tiglium* is considered as the only species possessed of cathartic properties.

The seeds of the *Croton tiglium* were formerly used in Europe under the name of Molucca grains; they were afterwards neglected, and it is only since Dr Whitelaw Ainslie called the attention of the profession to them, that they have again been employed by European practitioners. As the following observations by Dr White seem valuable, I shall quote them at full length.

"Take the seeds of the *Croton tiglium*, after having been each enveloped in a small ball of fresh cow-dung, about the size of a sparrow's egg, put them on some burning charcoal, and allow them to remain till the cow-dung is burnt or toasted dry, then remove them, and taking off carefully the shells from the seeds, pound the nuclei, and divide into pills, making two out of each grain; two, or at most three of which are a sufficient dose for an adult; half a drachm of honey, to two drachms of the mass proves a convenient medium for uniting it. The advantages derived from the above-mentioned process, are, in the first place, it facilitates the removal of the shell; secondly, it renders the nucleus more fit for pounding; and lastly, the gentle torrefaction it undergoes, corrects in a

great degree the natural acrimony of the nut. The Tamool, Canarese, and Sanscrit names of this nut, express its quality of liquefying the contents of the intestines. An intelligent *Ioqui* from Benares, tells me, that in his country, they boil the seeds soft in milk, stripping them first of their shells; after which they pound them, forming the mass by means of lime juice, at the rate of one pill from each seed; two of these making an ordinary dose. A mode in Guzerate is still more simple, consisting merely in pounding the kernels, without any previous operation, and forming, by means of honey, two pills from each nucleus, one of which generally suffices for a strong purge; at the same time directing a gill of warm water to be taken immediately after swallowing the pill: in this preparation the inherent acrimony of the kernel, makes up for the smallness of the dose, and the water drank above it ensures its speedy operation.

"The following directions are from a learned *Persee vydia*, of Surat.

"After having removed the shells from the seeds, tie the kernels in a small piece of cloth, like a bag; then put this into as much cow-dung-water as will cover the bag, and let it boil; secondly, when boiled, split the kernels in two, and take a small leaf (filament) ·from them, which is said to be poisonous; and thirdly, pound the whole into a mass, to which add two parts of *katha* (catechú), that is, to one drachm of croton, add two of *katha*, and divide into pills of two grains each; two of which are sufficient for one dose. The addition of the *katha* is said to correct its acrimony altogether, and to prevent any griping from ensuing."

The expressed oil which is obtained from the seeds, is now very much used in obstinate constipation, and in all cases in which it is necessary to evacuate the bowels with certainty and rapidity. In doses of from one to three drops, it operates as a drastic purgative; its operation is very rapid, generally in about an hour or two after the dose has been swallowed. From the smallness of the dose, it is admirably adapted for maniacs, or for persons labouring under temporary delirium; it is not admissible in very weak habits, nor ought it to be given to children nor to pregnant women. Dr Ainslie mentions that it has been used with success as an emmenagogue.

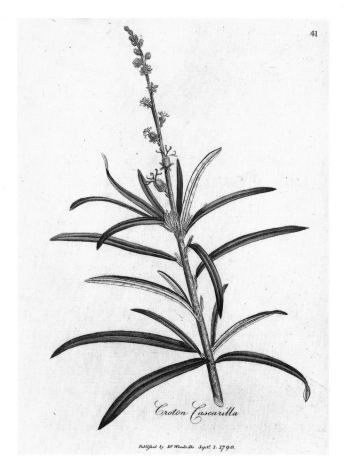

Croton Cascarilla

Published by Dr Woodville Sept.r 1. 1790.

CATHARTIC CROTON

CASCARILLA BARK TREE

Croton eleutheria

Class and Order, Monœcia Monadelphia. Nat. Ord. Euphorbiaceæ.
Gen. Char. Male Flowers; *Calix* cylindrical, of five segments; *Corolla* five petals; *Stamens* ten to fifteen. Female flowers; *Calix* five, on many segments; *Corolla* wanting; *Styles* three, bifid; *Capsule* three-celled, three-seeded.

A NATIVE of the Bahama and West Indian islands, growing in dry stony places; it is a low tree, seldom exceeding twenty feet in height, its stem and branches are thickly covered with whitish-grey mealy lichens, interspersed with numerous species of Opegrapha and other minute fungi. Its leaves are entire, somewhat cordate, elongated towards the apex, upper surface deep green, beneath silvery; flowers small, in axillary and terminal spikes.

The drug Cascarilla is imported in small quills, which are on the exterior white or light-grey, within of a pale cinnamon colour, and it possesses an agreeable aromatic flavour; it has been used in Europe ever since the year 1693. Like other newly introduced drugs, it was at first held in the highest esteem, then sank into almost total neglect.

Cascarilla is aromatic, stimulant, and tonic. It was at one time considered as possessing febrifuge virtues equal to cinchona, but experience has not substantiated its claims. When combined with cinchona, it is said to increase its efficacy, and at the same time to diminish its disagreeable taste. When burnt, it gives out an agreeable odour resembling that of musk; it is sometimes smoked, either alone or mixed with tobacco. When used alone, it increases the rapidity of the pulse and the heat of the surface, and causes a degree of mental excitement which is not followed by languor. Mixed with tobacco, it lessens its sedative and nauseating effects.

WHITE-BARKED CANELLA

Canella alba

Class and Order, Dodecandria Monogynia. Nat. Ord. Meliceæ.
Gen. Char. *Calix* three-lobed; *Petals* five; *Anthers* sixteen, adnate; *Nectarium* pitcher-shaped; *Berry* one-celled; *Seeds* two or four.

THE *Canella alba* forms a tree, standing from ten to fifteen feet in height; its leaves are of a deep shining green above, glaucous beneath, entire, obtuse, of a thick substance like those of laurel; flowers at the extremity of the branches, small, violet-coloured, and but seldom expanding, being fleshy, smooth, black, and shining.

This species is common to many of the West Indian islands and South America; it is likewise said to be one of the largest trees growing on Terra del Fuego, attaining, on that inhospitable shore, the height of fifty feet or upwards. The bark, which is the officinal part, is aromatic, as, indeed, is the whole plant; it is of a light greyish colour, but when the epidermis is removed, it is then of a very pale yellow-brown, in which state it is imported into this country, commonly rolled into quills. The specimens figured on the accompanying plate are represented with the epidermis attached; this is usually removed by a file or rasp. The bark of the older stems have a purplish hue on the exterior, but the liber is whiter than that of the younger branches.

Canella is an aromatic stimulant of considerable energy; it is rarely used by itself, but enters

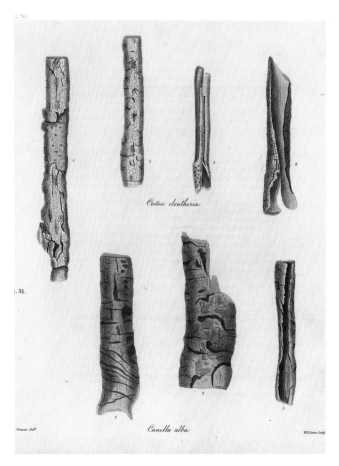

Croton eleutheria.

Canella alba.

CASCARILLA BARK TREE AND WHITE-BARKED CANELLA

into several officinal preparations, and is a useful addition to some bitters which are apt to cause nausea unless combined with an aromatic. The odour and taste of Canella are very similar to nutmeg.

COMMON WORMWOOD

Artemisia absinthium

Class and Order, Syngenesia Superflua. Nat. Ord. Compositæ.
Gen. Char. *Involucre* ovate or rounded, imbricated; *Receptacle* naked or hairy; *Florets* of the ray awl-shaped; *Pappus* none.

Root perennial and fibrous; stems round, channelled, growing two or three feet high, bearing at their extremities numerous drooping panicles of dull-yellow flowers; leaves bi-pinnatifid; the floral ones mostly entire. All Britain's native species of Artemisia appear to possess properties identical with the present plant, only differing in the greater or lesser degree of bitterness for which all the family are proverbial, but for medical purposes this alone is worth the attention of the practitioner.

Wormwood has a nauseous smell, and an extremely bitter taste; it is stimulant, tonic, and anthelmintic; and is applied to bruises to prevent discoloration; cataplasms made with its infusion are often useful in gangrenous and putrid sores. It contains an essential oil, which has the nauseous smell of the plant. The extract is merely a simple bitter, and has not the disagreeable odour.

ASARABACCA

Asarum europæum

Class and Order, Dodecandria Monogynia. Nat. Ord. Aristolochiæ.
Gen. Char. *Perianth* single, three cleft, superior; *Capsule* six-celled.

This species grows in woods in the north of England and is much sought after by medical men. From the crown of the perennial root, the leaves grow out in pairs on long foot-stalks, and from the axil of these springs the solitary flower, which is of a lurid purple, drooping, and of a coriaceous texture. The whole plant attains only a few inches in height; the leaves are of a full

bright green, and afford a good example of a reniform leaf. It produces its large but inconspicuous flower in May, which often continues on the stems till the fall of the year. Five species are mentioned in Loudon's Hortus Britannicus, all of which are natives of North America except the present plant.

The root of the Asarum is one of the most powrful errhines which we possess, the leaves also are sternutatory, but are much milder than the root. Given internally in doses of forty or fifty grains it causes vomiting and purging; the alcoholic tinctures are said to act in this way, but the extracts made by inspissating them act only as emetics. Aqueous decoctions and extracts are said to have neither purgative nor emetic properties, but to possess diuretic, diaphoretic, and emmenagogue virtues. It would seem from this statement, that the purgative and emetic qualities depend on a volatile principle, but as chemists have found a fixed active principle (*Cytisine*), which acts energetically both as an emetic and purgative, the statements above-noticed must be looked upon as partly imaginary.

MOUNTAIN ARNICA

Arnica montana

Class and Order, Syngenesia Superflua. Nat. Ord. Compositæ.
Gen. Char. *Receptacle* naked; *Pappus* simple; *Calix* with equal leaves; *Florets* of the ray generally with five filaments without anthers.

A hardy perennial, common to the mountainous parts of Europe, preferring moist shady situations. Stems about a foot high, roundish, rough, and hairy; flowers large, shewy, each on a separate stalk; of a full yellow, or dull gold colour; roots leaves oval, narrowing at their bases; cauline leaves sessile.

This species, which is often called leopardsbane, (a name applied to a nearly allied genus, *Doronicum*), is of easy culture, and increases readily by its roots; the flowers sometimes are of a brownish, and at others of a greenish hue. Four species are enumerated.

When given in small doses, the flowers of the *Arnica* are stimulant, emmenagogue, and antiseptic. In large doses, they give rise to anxiety, vertigo, vomiting, and purging, and even to coma. In countries where the plant is indigenous, infusions of all parts of it are popular remedies in internal contusion, in concussion of the brain, &c. In Germany, several authors of eminence have recommended the exhibition of the flowers in remittent and intermittent fevers, and in paralytic affections. Neumann of Dresden says that he has cured cataract by the internal use of the *Arnica*, but he at the same time used a collyrium, containing acetate of ammonia, in union with the *Arnica*. This plan of treatment I should not think deserving of repetition, as it seems founded on no rational plan. Rheumatism, inflammation of the kidneys, and a variety of other diseases of completely opposite characters, are said to have yielded to the use of this plant. The root and leaves are powerful errhines, especially when fresh. The root acts in the same way as the flowers when given internally, but is more energetic. It was at one time supposed to owe its medicinal properties to the presence of *Stychnia*; but Chevalier and Lassaigne have discovered a proximate vegetable principle, analogous to, or identical with, *Cytisine*, which was first obtained from the Laburnum, and which I have before mentioned as having been found by me in the broom, (*Cytisus scoparium*).

ELECAMPANE

Inula helenium

Class and Order, Syngenesia Superflua. Nat. Ord. Compositæ.
Gen. Char. *Involucre* imbricated, its scales spreading, outer ones especially, foliaceous; *Anthers* with bristles at their base; *Receptacle* naked; *Pappus* simple: *Flowers* yellow.—*Hooker.*

Elecampane is occasionally found growing wild in various parts of the British islands; is a hardy perennial, and readily increases by its roots, which are thick and large. The stems grow from three to five feet high, round, leafy and branching at the top; leaves large, ovate, slightly serrated, green above, hoary beneath, those on the stalks sessile and embracing the stem, the radical ones frequently a foot or more in length, growing on petiols; flowers large, terminal, of a full yellow colour. This species is found in most parts of Europe.

Elecampane root has a pleasant aromatic odour, and a bitterish, tough not unpleasant

taste; it is tonic, emmenagogue, diuretic, and sudorific. It is given in the form of powder, of decoction, and of vinous tincture. Little use is made of it by medical practitioners.

WHEAT

Triticum hybernum

Class and Order, Triandria Digynia. Nat. Ord. Gramineæ.
Gen. Char. "*Calix* two-valved, many-flowered, valves opposite, transverse, the sides (not the back) of one of them directed to the rachis, nearly equal; *Corolla* two-valved, valves lanceolate, exterior one accuminate or awned at the extremity; interior one bifid at the point."—*Hooker.*

This well-known plant, so universally cultivated, is supposed to have originally been introduced into Europe from Asia; but, from long culture, is most probably so altered in its appearance as not to be recognised in its native state. There are a considerable variety of kinds in general cultivation; the one retained in the modern pharmacopœias is known to agriculturists as the winter or Lammas wheat, and contains a larger proportion of starch than any of the others.

Wheat bread forms a large proportion of the food of both the higher and lower classes. In the Highlands of Scotland, in Wales, and some of the English counties, oat and barley bread form a principal part of the food of the poorer classes, and wheaten bread is looked upon as a luxury, rather than as a necessary of life. This is particularly the case in some of the more remote of the Highland counties of Scotland. Bread is made by kneading the flour into a stiff paste with water; yeast, or some other ferment, is then added, and the fermentation is allowed to proceed to a certain point. During the fermentation a quantity of carbonic acid gas is evolved, the toughness of the paste prevents its escape, and the heat of the oven expands it, and in this way the bread is rendered light and spongy. The oven is heated to about 490°F. A quantity of muriate of soda is added to the mass of dough to render it sapid. The various qualities of bread show, that, though the process is extremely simple in theory, it requires both attention and experience to carry it into practice successfully. Various adulterations are practised in the manufacture of this article; some of such magnitude as to have called for the attention of the legislature at various times. The adulterations are of various sorts. Some are intended to make a coarse flour assume the appearance of the finest; for this purpose alum is used. Others to increase the weight; among the most prevalent of these is the admixture of bone dust. The most curious adulteration with which I am acquainted is that mentioned by Professor Christison in his work on poisons, as having been very common in France. I shall quote the article at full length:

"A singular variety of adulteration with copper has lately been brought into public notice on the continent,—namely, the impregnation of bread with the sulphate of copper, which is used in small quantity for promoting the fermentation of the dough. This practice was first detected in some of the towns of Flanders, but has also been since found to prevail in France. Some chemists of reputation have indeed doubted altogether the existence of the practice; and *M. Barruel* in particular, who was consulted on the subject by the Profecture of Paris, has publicly declared his disbelief, because he remarked that, instead of favouring the panary fermentation, a very small proportion of sulphate of copper actually impeded it, and besides gave the bread a greenish colour of such depth that no customer would take it for a wholesome article. Subsequent inquiries, however, have shown that Barruel must have allowed himself to be misled, probably by using too much of the sulphate of copper. For the bakers of St Omer have admitted that they practice this adulteration for the sake of saving their yeast, the proportion required being an ounce of the salt in two pints of water for every hundred weight [*quintal*] of dough, or about an 1800th part. And it appears from an interesting set of experiments by *M. Meylink*, a chemist of Deventer, that, contrary to the statements of Barruel, sulphate of copper not only possesses the property of promoting the panary fermentation, but likewise constitutes in several important respects a source of adulteration, which ought to be prohibited and strictly looking after. He found that when he added to half a Flemish pound of dough from one grain to eight grains of sulphate of copper, fermentation took place more quickly than in the same dough without such addition, and nearly in proportion to the quantity of the salt used;—that the adulterated loaves when taken out of the oven were much better raised, and the loaf with only one grain of the salt likewise much whiter, than those which were not adulterated;—that a slight increase, however, in the proportion rendered the loaf greenish, and gave it a peculiar taste;—but especially that the employment of the salt of copper even in the small proportion of one grain had the singular effect of bringing about the complete fermentation of the dough with considerably less loss of weight than occurs in the common process of baking, the loss in the sound and in the adulterated loaves being in the proportion of 116 to 100. It certainly seems fully proved, then, that the adulteration of bread with sulphate of copper is an important fraud in more ways than one. Some doubt may be entertained whether any injury can result to the human body from even the habitual use of so small a quantity as is employed by the bakers; and, at all events, we may be satisfied that if any bad effects do result, this can only happen from the continual use of the adulterated bread for a great length of time. But there can be no doubt that the practice is a serious fraud on the public, by enabling the baker to make his loaves of the standard weight with a less allowance of nutritive material."

Carbonate of ammonia is also extensively used in the preparation of bread, but it is hardly to be looked upon as an adulteration. Potatoes and potatoe starch are also employed. Bread is sometimes used in the form of cataplasm made either with milk or water. A pleasant drink is made by infusing toasted bread in hot water; it is much used by dyspeptic persons, and in fevers and inflammatory diseases. Wheat-flour contains a much larger quantity of gluten than the flour of any other grain; to this it owes its superior nutritious properties.

CULTIVATED OAT

Avena sativa

Class and Order, Triandria Digynia. Nat. Ord. Gramineæ.
Gen. Char. *Panicle* lax; *Calix* two-valved, two-flowered; *Corolla* of two lanceolate valves, firmly enclosing the seed; exterior one bearing a twisted dorsal *awn*; upper florets often imperfect.—*Hooker.*

THE cultivated oat is an annual plant commonly grown on light soils; and the uses to which it is applied are too numerous and common to require notice in this place, as it falls under our

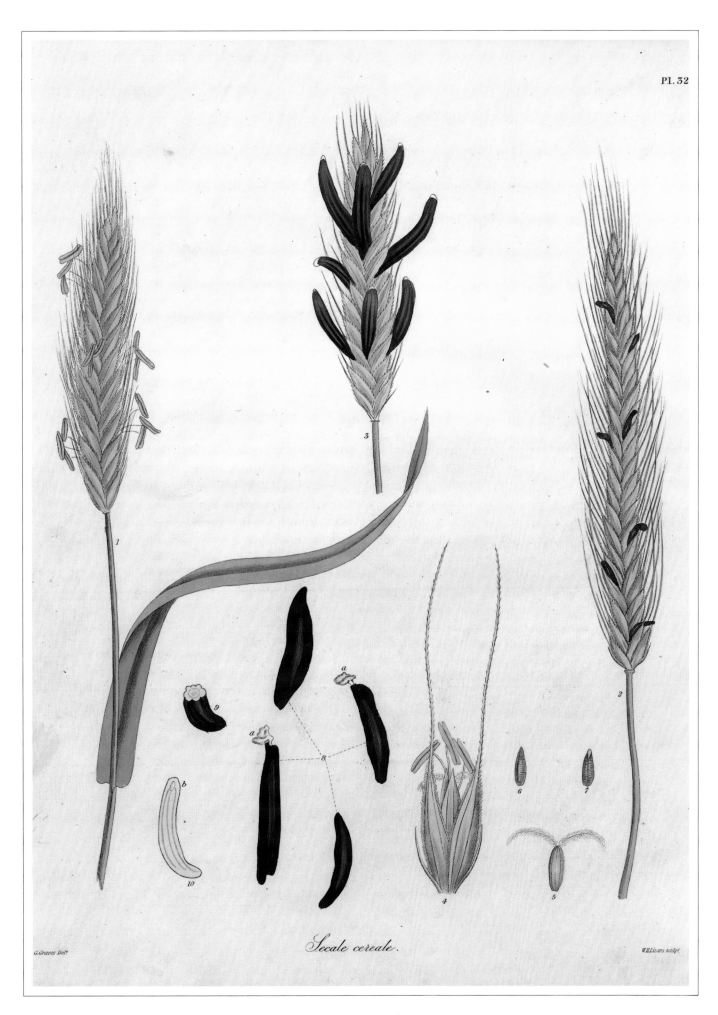

G. Graves Delt.

Secale cereale.

W. H. Lizars sculpt.

RYE

notice more as an article of food than medicine.

Its native country is unknown; but as it bears the cold of the more northern climates, it is probably indigenous to the colder parts of Europe. Nineteen species are enumerated by Loudon, besides a considerable number that have been transferred to the genus *Trisetum*.

The oat is much less nourishing than wheat. The meal boiled with water to the consistence of paste is much used in Scotland under the name of "porridge," and in some parts of England under the name of "burgou." Made into cakes, it forms the staple household bread in the north of Scotland. No yeast is used in the preparation of this bread; it is prepared by kneading the meal into a paste with cold water, and afterwards rolling it into thin circular pieces, which are fired on an iron plate hung over a common fire; no oven is ever used.

A decoction prepared from the ground grain is much used in febrile diseases as a diluent; it is known by the name of "gruel." Cataplasms made by boiling the meal in water to the consistence of paste are useful in phlegmonous inflammation, and in all cases in which such applications are indicated. Sinapisms are very easily and economically prepared by merely sprinkling the surface of such a cataplasm with mustard.

BARLEY

Hordeum distichon

Class and Order, Triandria Digynia. Nat. Ord. Gramineæ.

Gen. Char. *Calix* two-valved; *Valves* one-flowered, growing three together, the lateral one with anthers or pistils, intermediate ones perfect; *Corolla* two-valved.

BARLEY is considered to be a native of Tartary, and supports the rigours of the colder climates better than any other of the cereal grasses; and, in the more northern parts of Europe, is the only grain that can be cultivated. In such situations, its rapidity of growth is commensurate with the duration of their short-lived summers; being often sown and reaped in the short space of six weeks. Like wheat and oats, this plant consitutes a large portion of the food of the inhabitants where it grows, and its medical uses are of a secondary nature. The principal consumption of barley is for the purpose of malting, either for the use of the brewer or distiller.

Barley is used as aliment in various parts of France, in the Highlands of Scotland, and in the north of Europe. The bread prepared from it is less nourishing than that prepared from wheat. Whether taken in the form of bread or pottage, it acts on many persons as a gentle laxative, and is occasionally prescribed in cases of habitual constipation with that view. The decoction of barley, which is familiar to most persons under the name of "barley water," is an excellent diluent in fevers, and inflammatory diseases; it is a valuable remedy in diarrhœa, where there is a deficiency of the natural mucous secretion, or when an acrid secretion has supplied its place.

The process of malting is this: The grain is soaked in water till it become soft, and till the water acquire a reddish colour. It is then taken out and allowed to drain; when sufficiently drained, it is laid in a heap, and allowed to remain for about fifteen or sixteen hours, by which time, if the soaking has been properly conducted, it will begin to push out radicles; it must then be turned over frequently, to prevent the growth of the blade. It may be allowed to remain thus for about forty hours. It is then spread out to a depth not exceeding five inches, and constantly turned for forty-eight hours; by this means the grain is cooled and dried, is rendered of easy separation from the husk, and of greater solubility. It is now put into heaps, which are allowed to heat till the temperature is raised as high as the hand can bear; this generally takes place in about thirty hours. It is then again turned over and cooled, and lastly laid on a kiln and dried. Upon this part of the process depends the colour and name of the liquor afterwards prepared from it. For making ale, the malt is only dried; for making porter, the drying is carried so far as partly to roast the grain. The operation of brewing is exceedingly simple. The malt is digested for two or three hours in hot water, and this is repeated till the greater part of the soluble part is extracted. Hops are added at this part of the process if required. The united infusions are then boiled to the requisite strength, cool yeast is added, and the fermentation allowed to proceed to a certain length; the liquid is then put into casks, and allowed to remain there for some time, before being bottled or drawn off for use. Though the process is simple, yet the modifications are very numerous, and a great deal depends upon very slight variations, as the different qualities of the porter, ale, &c. from different breweries will sufficiently prove. In preparing malt spirit the first steps of the process are nearly the same as in brewing. When the fermentation has reached the proper point, the wort (that is the fermenting infusion of the malt) is run into the still, heat is applied, and the distillation is carried on till nearly all the spirit has run over; the first portion, which is fiery, and the last, which is weak, are united and reduced to a proper strength. In this way, Whisky and Usquebagh, the national spirits of Scotland and Ireland, are prepared. In both countries an inferior spirit is made from unmalted grain; the greater part of that made in Scotland is sent to the English market, where it is manufactured into gin.

RYE

Secale cereale

Class and Order, Triandria Digynia. Nat. Ord. Gramineæ.
Gen. Char. *Spikelets* in each tooth of the rachis solitary, two or three-flowered; the two lower florets fertile, sessile, opposite, the upper abortive; *Glumes* subulate, opposite, entire, shorter than the florets; lower *Paleæ* entire, with a very long bristle, upper bifid-toothed; *Scales* obovate, hairy; *Seed* coated, furrowed.

The rye falls under the notice of the medical practitioner from the circumstance of its producing the drug denominated *Ergot of Rye*; this substance is the seed in a state of disease, particularly common to a large variety of grasses. In the specimen figured on the annexed plate, will be observed one which I sowed, and after about two weeks it had swollen considerably, but no exterior sign of vegetation appeared; on cutting it lengthways, it appeared as if an attempt at vegetating had been made, but it was quite decayed. It two others the plumule had pushed out beyond the coating of the seed, but only formed a kind of fungous protuberance, which in a short time became quite putrid, with a peculiar odour, like decaying animal matter. In rye grown in Britain ergot rarely attains the size of our smallest specimen at fig. 8, but in American specimens, which we have been favoured with by the kindness of Mr Duncan, and also by Mr Lindsay, chemists of Edinburh, the size is as figured on the plate. The spike, fig. 1, is from Canada; fig.

3, with fine specimens of Ergot, from East Florida; and fig. 2. British.

In many parts of continental Europe, the rye forms a principal part of the food of the inhabitants; in some seasons and in particular districts the grain is subject to a disease which renders it highly poisonous to man and animals. Some animals do not seem easily affected by it; others, among which are swine, geese, fowls, &c. are affected with diarrhœa, vertigo, and latterly with suppurating tumours and gangrene. Two distinct diseases are caused by the habitual use of the ergotized grain. One, the *Ergotisme convulsive* of the French; the other, the *Gangrene sêche* of the same authors. The first form of the disease commences with vertigo, dimness of sight, and loss of feeling, followed by cramps and convulsions of the whole body, *risus sardonicus*, yellowness of the countenance, excessive thirst, excruciating pains in the limbs, and dull, small, and imperceptible pulse. When the symptoms are of this aggravated nature, the disease generally proves fatal in from twenty-four to forty-eight hours. In milder forms, the convulsions come on in paroxysms, and are preceded for some time by lassitude and the feeling of insects crawling on the surface of the body; in the intervals the appetite is voracious. The pulse and excretions are natural; the disease either

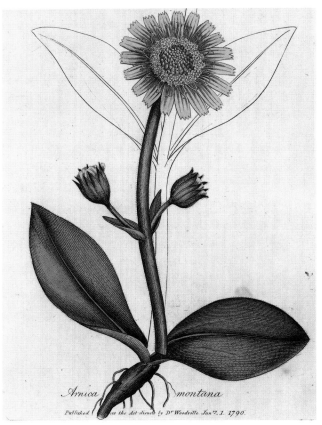

Arnica montana
Published for the Act directe by Dʳ Woodville Janʸ 1. 1790.

MOUNTAIN ARNICA

terminates in recovery, preceded by scattered suppurations, cutaneous eruptions, anasarca and diarrhœa, or it ends fatally amidst prolonged sopor and convulsions. The next form of the disease,—the dry gangrene, commences with general uneasiness, weakness, and a feeling of insects crawling over the skin. When these symptoms have continued for some days or weeks, the extremities become cold, stiff, white, and benumbed, and so insensible that deep incisions are not felt; excruciating pains supervene, with fever, headache and bleeding from the nose; finally, the affected parts gradually shrivel and drop off by the joints; healthy granulations succeed, but the system is frequently so worn out that the person dies before this favourable change occurs. The appetite continues voracious throughout. Various other modifications of this formidable epidemic have been observed in Germany and Switzerland. From the improved state of agriculture, the disease is becoming more rare, though some cases have occurred in Germany since the commencement of the present century. Another very peculiar property has been attributed to the ergot of rye; it is that of exciting the action of the uterus when dormant from protracted unsuccessful efforts to expel the child. This property is supported by the testimony of many accoucheurs; but it is a remedy which ought to be given only in urgent cases, and in the most careful and guarded manner. It has been said to have the power of causing abortion; but it is the opinion of the best authorities, that it only possesses the property of increasing the action of the uterus when it has already commenced, and that it has no power of inducing uterine action in the early months of pregnancy, at least not without causing constitutional disturbance of a very dangerous nature. The cause of the ergot is not ascertained; it is by some supposed to arise from the puncture of an insect, by others it is said to arise from the presence of parasitic fungi.

MEADOW SAFFRON

Colchicum autumnale

Class and Order, Hexandria Trigynia. Nat. Ord. Melanthaceæ.

Gen. Char. *Perianth* single, tubular, very long, rising from a spathe; *Limb* campanulate, six-parted, petaloid; *Capsule* three-celled; *Cells* united at the base.

Bulb solid, gibbous, outer skin dry, smooth, deep chestnut colour; beneath this, the fleshy coat is covered with a thin pellicle of a bright brown, with parallel lines; a deep groove, commencing at the base of the root, extends its whole length, along which the flowers ascend; leaves long, plane sheathing, the inner ones narrower; tube white, very long, narrow, often exceeding six inches in length, surrounded at the base with a membranous sheath; stamens inserted into the segments of the flower; germen situated at the base of the bulb; styles continuing the whole length of the tube; capsule of three cells, united at the base; seeds round and flattened.

Few of Britain's native plants have a more curious mode of fructification than the meadow saffron; towards the close of autumn, its delicate purple flowers appear and expand in succession, continuing in blossom for some weeks; when this is past, the flowers become dry and withered, but do not fall off until the following year. The leaves appear early in the spring, and with them arises the fruit-stalk, bearing on its summit two or three capsules; those in the young state are situated on the crown of the young bulb, as at figure 3, and remain quite dormant during winter. With the advancing year, the leaves and stem elongate, and the styles, which were persistent on the germen, show a tendency to decay, and before the capsules emerge from the ground are entirely withered. The capsules continue enlarging, and the stem increasing in length with the leaves, until they arrive at maturity, when they are nearly the size of a pigeon's egg. The seeds ripen about June or July, when the leaves assume a pale hue, and in a few weeks afterwards entirely disappear; the bulb which produced them is then dry and hard, but does not perish the same year, so that each bulb may be correctly called a biennial.

The roots possess but little of their active properties during the autumn, but in the spring and summer are in their greatest vigour, and should be dug up for use and quickly dried.

Colchicum is found in moist meadowland. It grows readily in gardens, with double white as well as purple flowers; and some that I had occasion to examine in the month of December last, and from which part of the accompanying figures were drawn, were as acrid as I ever met with them.

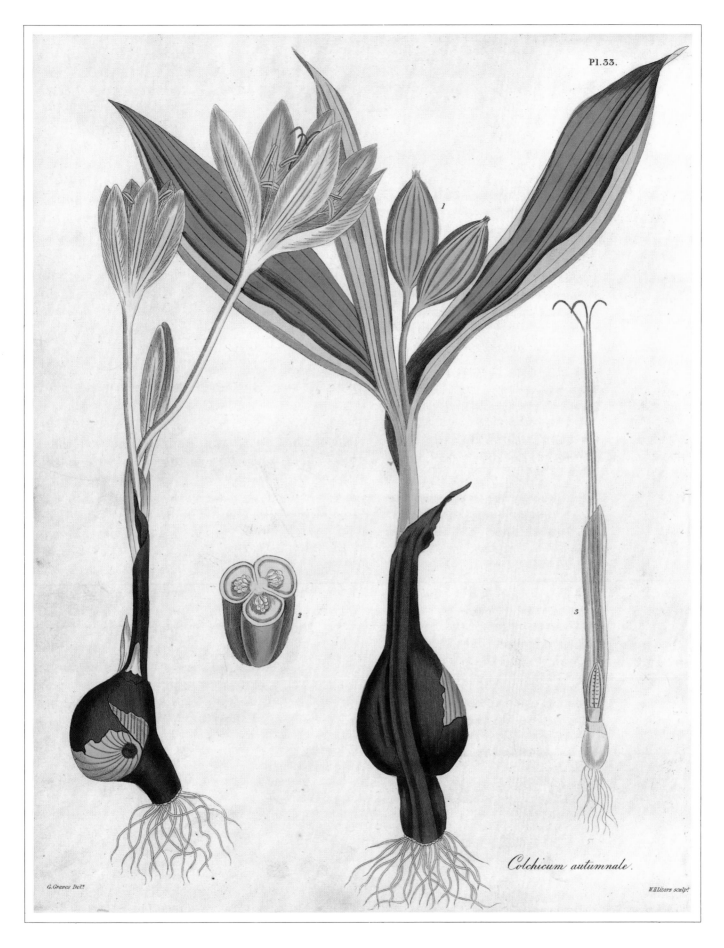

Pl.33.

Colchicum autumnale.

G.Graves Delt.

W.H.Lizars sculpt.

MEADOW SAFFRON

The bulb of the Colchicum, when fresh, contains a milky viscid juice, which possesses extreme acridity, inflaming the mouth, tongue, and fauces when applied to them, and causing considerable irritation of the mucous membrane. When taken into the system, various effects are produced, depending both on the quantity given, and on the constitution of the person who takes it. In small doses, it usually acts as a diuretic, and with this view it has been strongly recommended by Stoerk and other German authors in anasarca, hydrothorax, &c. In somewhat larger doses, it acts both as a sedative and cathartic. In cases in which small doses have been continued for a length of time, and where their effects have been allowed to accumulate, symptoms of the most violent nature, such as vomiting, colic, purging, sometimes of blood, tremors, cold sweats, faining, and delirium, present themselves, and several fatal cases are recorded. In some constitutions, even an ordinary dose may give rise to unpleasant symptoms; it is therefore necessary to observe caution in prescribing it. A good deal of controversy has taken place with regard to the specific action of Colchicum in gout and rheumatism; but it is now generally admitted on all hands, that, whatever the nature of its action may be, its effects, under judicious management, are highly beneficial. Some attribute the good effects of Colchicum in the above-named diseases to its sedative properties; others to its cathartic, supposing that the irritation which it causes in the mucous membrane of the intestines diminishes the inflammatory action going on in the mucous membrane of the joints, on the principle of counter-irritation.

Colchicum possesses the remarkable property of increasing the quantity of uric acid in the urine. Every part of the meadow saffron is active, but the bulb and seeds are the parts commonly employed in medicine.

WHITE HELLEBORE

Veratrum album

Class and Order, Polygamia Monœcia. Nat. Ord. Melanthaceæ.
Gen. Char. Fertile Flower; *Calix* wanting; *Corolla* of six petals; *Stamens* six; *Ovaries* three; *Capsules* three, many-seeded.
Male Flower; same as fertile, but no ovaries.

A hardy plant, a native of Italy, Switzerland, Austria, and Russia, and is now commonly met with in gardens. The root is perennial, thick, with numerous fibres; stems strong, round, upright, hairy, attaining to three or four feet high; leaves numerous, large, oval, entire, plaited, sessile: flowers pale green, in long branched spikes, the perfect and male flowers interspersed. The properties of the species appear identical, and they are all of easy cultivation.

The medicinal properties of the Veratrum are similar to those of the Colchicum. Its activity is greater, and many cases of poisoning with it are recorded. Dr Christison quotes from Rust's Journal the following account: "A family of eight people, in consequence of eating bread for a whole week, in which the powder of the root had been introduced by mistake instead of cummin seeds, were attacked with pains in the belly, a sensation as if the whole intestines were wound up in a clue, swelling of the tongue, soreness of the mouth, and giddiness; but they all recovered by changing the bread and taking gentle laxatives." Dr Christison again quotes from Horn's Archives. "Three people took the root by mistake for Galanga root. The symptoms that ensued were very characteristic of its double action. In an hour they had all burning in the throat, gullet, and stomach, followed by nausea, dysuria, and vomiting; weakness and stiffness of the limbs; giddiness, blindness, and dilated pupil; great faintness; convulsive breathing; and small pulse. One of them, an elderly woman, who took the largest share, had an imperceptible pulse, stertorous breathing, and total insensibility, even to ammonia held under her nose. Next day she continued lethargic, complained of headache, and had an eruption like flea-bites."

CATECHU

Acacia catechu

Class and Order, Polygamia Monœcia. Nat. Ord. Leguminosæ.
Gen. Char. Hermaphrodite Flower; *Calix* five-toothed; *Corolla* of five petals; *Stamens* from four to one-hundred; *Pistil* one; *Legume* of two valves.
Male Flower; *Calix* five-toothed; *Corolla* of five petals; *Stamens* four to one-hundred.

This species forms a low bushy tree, from twelve to twenty feet high. The stem is covered with rough brown bark; leaves placed alternately on the younger branches, composed of from fifteen to thirty pinnæ; the pinnulæ of about forty pairs, the partial pinnæ about two inches long; spines short, recurved, situated in pairs at the base of each leaf; flowers in long dense spikes, arising from the axillæ of the leaves; corolla of one piece, divided into five segments or petals; stamens twice the length of the corolla.

The plants forming the genus Acacia were separated by Willdenow from the genus Mimosa, in which they were placed by Linnæus, and from which they differ in the form of the seed-pods, which in the true Mimosa separate into one-seeded joints, and the flowers are furnished with but eight stamens.

It is an extensive genus, all the species of which are natives of the warmer parts of the old and new continent. Loudon enumerates eighty-two species. They mostly require the protection of a greenhouse, though two or three species thrive and produce their flowers in the open air.

Catechu is one of the most powerful astringents which we possess. It is also safe, and may be used in almost all cases in which astringents are indicated. Duncan's Dispensatory states:

"Catechu has the appearance of a dried extract of various forms, rounded masses, or cut into squares or lozenges. It is perfectly opaque, and has always an earthy fracture."

From the large quantity of tannin which catechu contains, it has been proposed to use it in the preparation of leather; though the expense of importing, and the price of the drug itself, would prevent its being used in Europe, yet in India there is no doubt that it might be successfully employed. The tannin of catechu differs in some of its less important properties from pure tannin.

OFFICIAL SPURGE

Euphorbia officinarum

Class and Order, MONŒCIA MONANDRIA. NAT. ORD. EUPHORBIACEÆ.

Gen. Char. *Involucre* of one petal including several barren flowers and one fertile. Sterile flower; a single *Stamen*, without calix or corolla. Fertile flower; a single *Pistil*, without calix (or rarely a very minute one) or corolla; *Germen* three-lobed; *Styles* three-cleft; *Capsule* three-seeded.

THE structure of the flowers of this genus appears to have been formerly very imperfectly understood, but it has been recently fully investigated, and the details, as given in the generic character, clearly ascertained. In structure there is a considerable affinity with that of *Reseda*, the Mignonette.

All the species of this numerous tribe abound in a milky acrid juice, which corrodes the skin wherever it comes in contact with it. The officinal species is a native of Africa, but thrives in hot-houses. The stem grows to the height of four or five feet, sometimes branched at the summit, at others simple, with six to eight angles, which, in the younger branches, are caused by deep furrows, which become nearly obsolete as the plant advances in age. Flowers solitary, sparingly produced on the edges of the ridges; yellowish-green; the stem is leafless.

The whole family are possessed of similar properties. Our native ones, though small, are indued with very energetic properties, and are often applied to eat off warts.

Dr Duncan describes the mode of collecting the Euphorbium resin thus: "The inhabitants of the lower regions of Atlas make incisions in the branches of the plant with a knife, a corrosive milky juice issues, which after being heated by the sun, becomes a substance of a whitish yellow colour, and in the month of September, drops off and forms *Euphorbium*. The plants produce abundantly only once in four years, but this fourth year's produce is more than all Europe can consume, for, being a very powerful cathartic, it is but little used. The people who collect Euphorbium are obliged to tie a cloth over their mouth and nostrils, to prevent the small dusty particles from annoying them, as they produce incessant sneezing. The branches are used in tanning morocco leather, and the juice is in great request among the women as a depilatory." Euphorbium is an acrid and drastic purgative; it is never, or very seldom, used internally. Applied to the skin, it causes increased heat and redness. Dr Christison mentions fatal cases,—one occurred under his own observation in the Royal Infirmary of Edinburgh, and was supposed to have been caused by a mixture containing Euphorbium having been taken, which was intended to cure horses of the grease. Dr C. says, the symptoms of poisoning with Euphorbium in man are violent griping and purging, with burning heat of the throat and fauces, followed by exhaustion. The appearances after death are, highly inflamed state of the stomach, which is sometimes covered with gangrenous spots.

WHITE MUSTARD

Sinapis alba

Class and Order, Tetradynamia Siliquosa. Nat. Ord. Cruciferæ.
Gen. Char. *Pod* nearly round, with nerved valves; *Style* small; short, acute; *Seeds* disposed in one series; *Calix* spreading.

This common plant is found among rubbish, and in neglected and uncultivated places; its hispid pods and pinnated leaves distinguish it from the following species. It is cultivated as a salad, and eaten when the seed leaves only have appeared; its seeds are much larger than those of the black mustard, but less pungent in their taste, though often mixed in the manufacture of flour of mustard. Its properties are similar to those of the other species, but less active.

BLACK MUSTARD

Sinapis nigra

Class and Order, Nat. Ord. and Generic Character, see S. Alba.

This species is found under hedges and in waste places, growing from one to three feet high, and is readily distinguished from the preceding species by its seed-vessel and large lower leaves. Black mustard is extensively cultivated for its seed, from which the well-known condiment mustard is procured.

Under the name of "Flour of Mustard," the powder of the seeds is familiar to all. Its uses as a condiment are also well known. The French mustard is much weaker than that used in England; this arises from the mode of preparation. In France the seeds are merely reduced to powder; in Britain they are first submitted to pressure, by which a quantity of bland fixed oil is expressed, and the cake which remains, is rendered much more pungent. Though the process be so well known in this country, yet in France it was considered necessary to have recourse to M. Robinet, a celebrated chemist, to verify it by experiment.

Mustard possesses tonic, emetic, and rubefacient properties. When prescribed as a tonic, the seeds are directed to be swallowed in their entire state. In dyspepsia, arising from languid action of the stomach, and that torpid state of the intestinal canal which frequently accompanies paralysis, they are often beneficial. The flour of mustard mixed with water has been long used as an emetic by the common people. In that species of asphyxia which is caused by the choke-damp of coal mines, a mustard emetic is the common remedy, and generally succeeds in rousing the person from the torpor in which he is plunged. I had an opportunity of trying it in a very great number of cases of cholera asphyxia and would still recommend it in the stage of diarrhœa, but not in the blue stage. Dr Lindsay also gave it in small doses as a diffusible stimulus, and from this mode of treatment I have seen very good effects. As a rubefacient, mustard is extremely valuable; where immediate counter-irritation is requisite, it is much superior to cantharides. In fever, where there is determination to the head, cataplasms of mustard (sinapisms) applied to the soles of the feet, and to the whole of the lower extremities, are often of great use. Care must be taken in the latter stages of fever that the sinapisms are not allowed to remain too long on, as gangrene has been known to supervene.

POMEGRANATE

Punica granatum

Class and Order, Icosandria Monogynia. Nat. Ord. Myrtaceæ.
Gen. Char. *Calix* of five segments; *Petals* five; *Berry* many-celled, many-seeded.

The pomegranate, from the earliest times, has been cultivated as a favourite fruit, particularly in the southern parts of Europe, in Arabia, in Persia, and in the Grecian Archipelago; it has been introduced into the East and West Indies, and the fruit produced in these latter countries is said to surpass in flavour that found in its native stations. In England it rarely rises to more than a shrub, but in its native country is said to form a tree eighteen or twenty feet in height; it produces a profusion of brilliant scarlet flowers, which in Britain is rarely succeeded by fruit; it sometimes varies with white, also with double flowers. "In its wild state it forms a thorny bush like our hawthorn." Only two species are recorded.

Pl.35.

Pl.34.

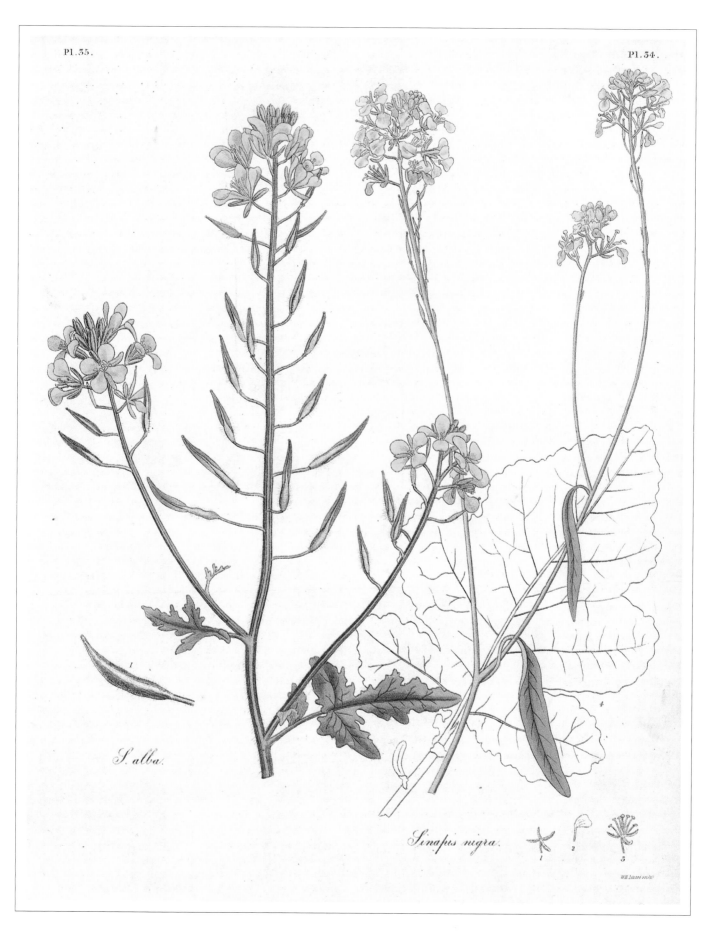

S. alba.

Sinapis nigra.

BLACK MUSTARD AND WHITE MUSTARD; FIG.1, CALIX; FIG.2, A PETAL; FIG.3, CALIX
AND STAMENS, PETALS REMOVED. A RIPE SEED-POD OF SINAPIS ALBA.

The pulp of the pomegranate is of a subacid sweetish taste, it allays heat, quenches thirst, and acts as a gentle aperient; it is particularly grateful in warm climates. The rind of the fruit is highly astringent, and where the fruit is abundant, this part of it is used in tanning. The flowers are frequently used, both internally and externally, as astringents. Of late the bark of the root has been much spoken of as a remedy in tape-worm.

"This remedy against tænia, known to the ancients, has been recently revived. It had been formerly employed and recommended by Mr P. Breton, according to Dr Chapotin. The following is his mode of exhibiting it. Take two ounces of the dried root of the pomegranate tree, boil them in two pints (*litres*) of water down to twelve ounces. Of this decoction sixty-four grammes (two ounces) to be given every half hour. The worm is often voided twelve hours after the first quantity has been taken. This practice may be repeated for four or five days successively, but must be suspended if the patient feels vertigos, an uneasy state and pains in the intestines. Castor oil is commonly given after the four draughts, even when the worm has been voided.

"It must be observed, that to obtain a constant success from this remedy, we must always use the bark of the root of the wild pomegranate, which grows in Africa, Spain, and in some provinces of the south of France.

"According to M. Bourgeoise, this remedy ought never to be administered until the patient has voided portions of tænia.

"For the introduction of pomegranate bark as a cure for the tape-worm, we are indebted to a Mussulman Fakir of Calcutta, who having in a few hours relieved an English gentleman in 1804, was prevailed on to disclose his secret, which was then communicated by Mr Russell for general information."

COLTSFOOT

Tussilago farfara

Class and Order, Syngenesia Superflua. Nat. Ord. Compositæ.
Gen. Char. *Involucre* formed of a single row of equal, linear scales; *Receptacle* naked; *Flowers* radiant; *Corollas* of the circumference long, linear, numerous, of the disk few; *Pappus* simple.

Coltsfoot is a common perennial plant, abounding in moist situations, and producing its blossoms among the earliest of Britain's native flowers; in mild seasons often as early as the end of February. Roots strongly creeping; flowers appearing before the leaves, at first erect, but after flowering, drooping; leaves large, deep-green, beneath thickly coated with a dense tomentum; these begin to appear as the flowers decay.

The leaves of this plant enter into the composition called Herb Tobacco, and in some parts of Britain the leaf-stalks are candied, and used to alleviate coughs and asthmatic affections.

Coltsfoot is recommended in phthisis and other pulmonary complaints, and in scrofula; but the benefit which is said to accure from its use ought to be attributed rather to the milk diet, with which it is generally prescribed, than to any inherent virtue. The flowers and leaves are both employed; the former have rather an agreeable odour and a weak bitter taste; the latter have a more bitter taste, and are highly spoken of by some authors as remedies in scrofula. Several quack medicines are prepared from this plant, and are extensively used in phthisis, asthma, and other affections.

COMMON SMALL-LEAVED ELM

Ulmus campestris

Class and Order, Pentandria Digynia. Nat. Ord. Ulmaceæ.
Gen. Char. *Perianth* single, superior, persistent, four or five-cleft; *Capsule* compressed, winged all round, one-seeded.

This well known tree grows to a large size, with rugged bark, and small leaves, the flowers grow in dense clusters; its value as a timber tree is great, as it is not subject to decay from excessive moisture. Before the introduction of iron pipes for the supplying of London and other large towns with water, elm ones were in general use for that purpose.

The medicinal virtues of the elm are so slight, that it might be expunged from the Materia Medica with great propriety. Decoctions of the inner bark have been occasionally recommended in dropsy and in ichthyosis. Klaproth discovered a peculiar principle in the elm, to which he gave the name of *Ulmine*; it exists in many other trees

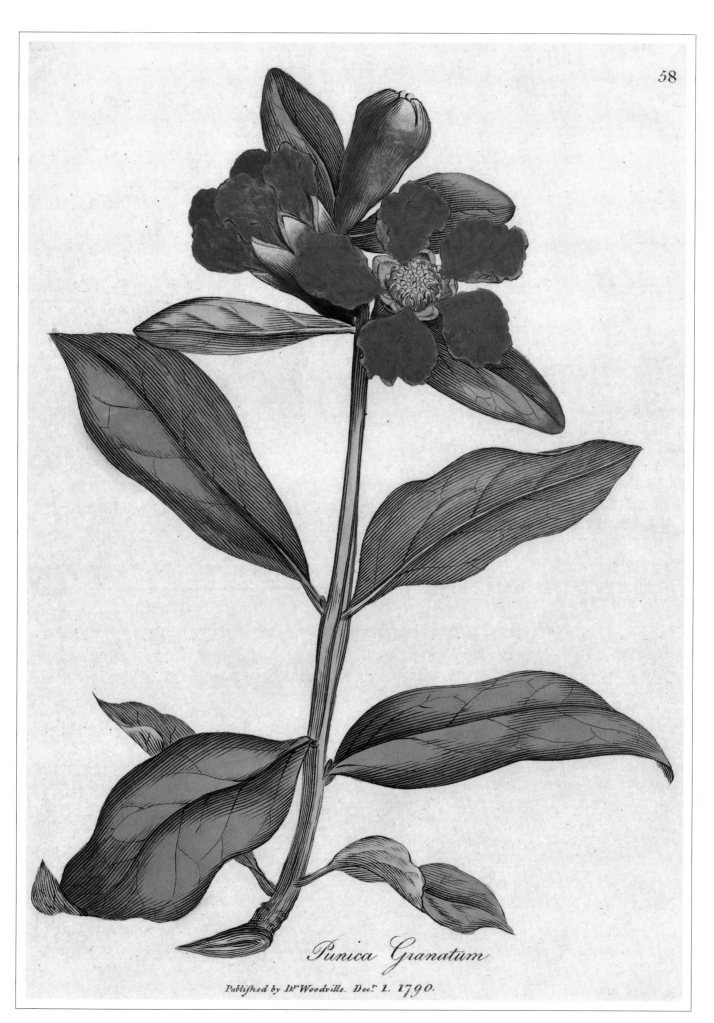

Punica Granatum

Published by Dr. Woodville. Decr. 1. 1790.

POMEGRANATE

and vegetables; it is solid, tasteless, inodorous, of a shining black colour; it is insoluble in cold water, and sparingly soluble in boiling, to which it imparts a yellow colour. It is soluble in alcohol and in sulphuric acid, it reddens litmus paper, and is very soluble in the alkalies.

Vauquelin, Berzelius, and other chemists have examined *Ulmine.*

COMMON ELDER

Sambucus nigra

Class and Order, Pentandria Trigynia. Nat. Ord. Caprifoliaceæ.
Gen. Char. *Calix* five-cleft; *Corolla* rotate, five-lobed; *Berry* inferior, three or four-seeded.

A common plant in coppices and hedgerows, forming a low tree. Its branches contain an unusual quantity of pith. The wood is hard, and was used for manufacturing musical instruments. Its rich purple berries are in much used for making into wine, but are in Ireland and Scotland held in disrepute. In Scotland, the elder is called *Boutrey* or *Bon-trey.* It varies with green berries, also in having deeply cut leaves. The last variety is called the parsley-leaved elder, and has been considered as a distinct species by several authors.

The flowers, leaves, and fruit of the elder are occasionally given internally. The flowers are most frequently used; they are considered stimulant, diaphoretic, and deobstruent. The inner bark of the young branches is sometimes prescribed as a purgative. The young leaf-buds are also cathartic, but their action is so violent as to render them unsafe as remedies. A syrup, prepared from the fruit, is in vogue in France as a gentle aperient and sudorific. Wine, having some resemblance to Frontignac, is prepared from the flowers, and is often sold under that appellation. The fruit, when taken in large quantity, is apt to cause nausea and vomiting; and in some constitutions a very small quantity acts as a pretty smart emetic. By distillation the flowers yield a volatile oil of the consistence of butter, having their flavour and other properties. The distilled water contains a perceptible quantity of ammonia.

COMMON BUCKTHORN

Rhamnus catharticus

Class and Order, Pentandria Monogynia. Nat. Ord. Rhamneæ.
Gen. Char. *Calix* campanulate, four or five-cleft; *Petals* four or five, or wanting; *Stamens* opposite the petals; *Berry* two or four-celled, two or four-seeded.

A low spreading shrub, not unfrequently met with in hedges and low woods; "leaves with four or six strong lateral nerves parallel with the margin or rib." In the perfect flowers the calix is urceolate. The berries in the unripe state yield a yellow dye, and in this state are known by the name of French berries; when ripe the juice is purple. The bark yields a beautiful yellow dye; its purgative properties are said to be communicated to the flesh of such birds as feed on its berries. The other native species, *R. frangula*, is also cathartic, and has dark purple berries, containing only two seeds, which before they are ripe, dye wool green and yellow, when ripe blue, blue-grey, and green. The wood, prepared as charcoal, is used by the makers of gunpowder. Twenty-four species are described.

The fruit of the *Rhamnus catharticus* was at one time a good deal used as a purgative; but, from the violence of its operation, and the disagreeable symptoms to which it gave rise, it has of late fallen into disuse. On the Continent it is still prescribed, chiefly in the form of syrup. When combined with lime and alumina, the juice of the berries forms the well-known pigment "sap-green." The inner bark is said to possess all the active properties of the fruit, and to be more apt to cause vomiting.

COMMON TORMENTIL

Tormentilla officinalis

Class and Order, Icosandria Polygynia. Nat. Ord. Rosaceæ.
Gen. Char. *Calix* of eight segments, alternately smaller; *Petals* four.

Root perennial, large, woody, exterior of a dark-brown, within of a bright-red, becoming more intense when growing in a dry soil; stems numerous, at first procumbent, then erect, branching upward, usually dichotomous; flowers of four petals, but often varying with five, even on the same stem. When it possesses five petals, it usually has ten segments to the calix, which are the essential characters by which the genus *Potentilla* is distinguished from this. By some authors the two genera are united, from the circumstance of the petals and calix not being constant in the number of their parts in either genus. It is to be regretted that the genera are still kept separate.

The Tormentil grows in abundance on moors, commons, and open woods; in the latter particularly, if shady, it is apt to become quite erect.

Tormentil root is one of the most powerful of the vegetable astringents. Dr Thomson says that it is only surpassed by catechu and nut-galls. Its taste is austere and somewhat aromatic, and it is one of the pleasantest of the native medicines of this class. As an external application, it has been recommended for the removal of warts. In leucorrhœa and in gonorrhœa, I have seen very good effects result from the use of the decoction as an injection. Internally, it is useful in chronic diarrhœas, and in all cases where astringents are indicated.

WILD PLUM-TREE

Prunus domestica

Class and Order, Icosandria Monogynia. Nat. Ord. Rosaceæ.
Gen. Char. *Calix* inferior, of five leaves; *Petals* five; *Fruit* a drupe containing a hard smooth nut.

This species or variety of plum is occasionally found in our woods and hedge-rows, and is esteemed by many botanists, together with *P. spinosa*, as a variety of *P. institia*; whether it is a species or not, it appears permanent. This, as well as the bullace, *P. institia*, is much less abundant than the sloe, *P. spinosa*.

The fruit of the *Prunus domestica* is sweet and sub-acid; it is not considered a very safe fruit when fresh, as, when taken in quantity, it frequently gives rise to cholic, diarrhœa, and other unpleasant symptoms. When dried they are called prunes. Though the fruit ripens easily, and grows both in England and Scotland, yet, as far as I am aware, no attempt was ever made to prepare prunes in either. The best are imported from France. In febrile and inflammatory diseases they are often given, as, in addition to their nutrient and demulcent properties, they act on the bowels as a gentle laxative. Intestinal concretions have been frequently found to have a prune stone for their nucleus.

SCOTCH FIR

Pinus sylvestris

Class and Order, Monœcia Monadelphia. Nat. Ord. Coniferæ.
Gen. Char. Barren flowers in crowded, racemose catkins; the scales peltate, bearing two one-celled, sessile anthers; *Perianth* none. Fertile flowers in an ovate catkin; its scales closely imbricated, two-flowered, perianth none; *Pericarp* one-seeded, terminated by a long, winged appendage, and covered with the imbricated scales, forming a cone or strobilus.

This, which is the only species of fir indigenous to the British islands, is found in abundance in the mountainous districts of Scotland, as well as in the northern parts of the continent of Europe; the trees growing on poor soil in elevated situations produce the most valuable timber; it grows to a vast size; Dr Hooker mentions having been shown a plank from the largest tree cut down in the Duke of Gordon's forests of Glenmore, that measured five and a-half feet in diameter. It is a valuable tree for its timber, as well as for the pitch, tar, and turpentine extracted from it; when planted in large masses it forms a noble object, but growing singly is unsightly, and often becomes stunted and deformed. The Highlands of Scotland have extensive natural forests of this species, and in such situations it is not only an object of much grandeur, but likewise of great utility.

NORWAY SPRUCE FIR

Pinus abies

Class and Order, Nat. Ord. and Gen. Char. See *Pinus sylvestris*.

The Norway Spruce Fir is one of the most valuable of the European forest trees, and frequently attains the height of one hundred and fifty feet or upwards; it is a native of the mountainous parts of Europe, and abounds in

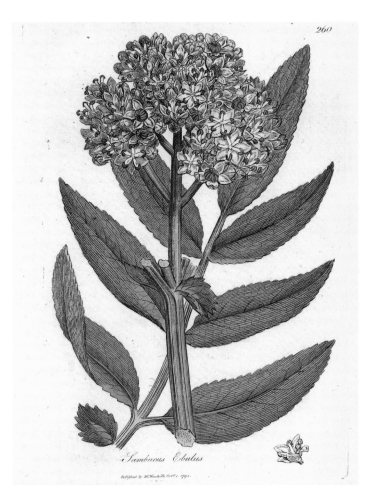

Sambucus Ebulus

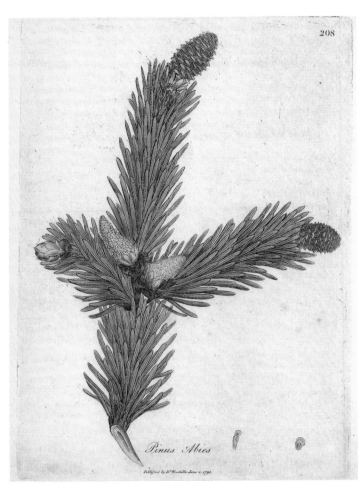

Pinus Abies

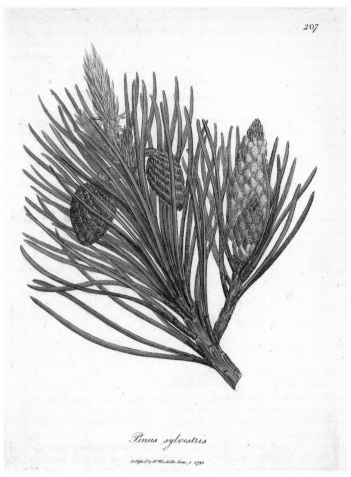

Pinus sylvestris

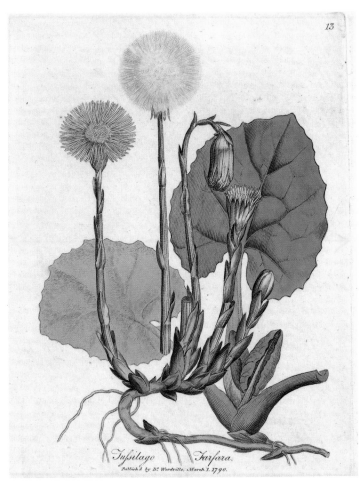

Tussilago Farfara

TOP LEFT: COMMON ELDER, TOP RIGHT: NORWAY SPRUCE FIR, BOTTOM LEFT:
SCOTCH FIR, BOTTOM RIGHT: COLTSFOOT

the northern provinces; it is of common occurrence in our plantations, and British grown timber is held in considerable estimation; but by far the greater part of that used for mechanical and domestic purposes is imported from the north of Europe. Though it grows readily in Britain, it never attains the size of those of Norway and Sweden; but it is by no means a small tree; it is highly ornamental, which, combined with its economic and pharmaceutic properties, renders it well deserving the attention of the forest planter.

BALM OF GILEAD FIR

Pinus balsamifera

Class and Order, Nat. Ord. and Gen. Char. See *Pinus sylvestris.*

THIS is a very elegant species, and in its native forests attains a great height. It abounds in the colder parts of North America, in lofty and exposed situations. The climate of Britain does not appear congenial to it, as it rarely forms a large tree, and seldom survives more than twenty or thirty years. It has a considerable resemblance to the silver fir, but its leaves are shorter, broader, and not so pointed. When its cones are at maturity, they exude considerable quantities of a resinous transparent fragrant fluid, as do the stems when wounded. This resin is the Canada balsam of the shops, and is often sold under the name of Balm of Gilead.

The following conspectus of the pine tribe by MM. Morington, Duponchel and Bonastre, is so comprehensive and useful, that I shall quote it at full length from Duncan's Dispensatory.

"Section I.—*Pines.*
"*Pinus maritima*—Sea pine—Pine of Landes—Sea-coasts of the south of Europe. Product: Turpentine of Bourdeaux; contains much volatile oil; employed much in the navy and in the arts; little esteemed in pharmacy.
"*Pinus sylvestris*—Scotch fir—North of Europe. Product: Tenacious thick resin, containing little oil; yields excellent tar, pitch, and *brais gras* for the navy.
"*Pinus rigida*—Rigid pine—Coast of Canada, very cold climate. Product: Resinous juice, said to be black; resin like the preceding.

"*Pinus australis* or *palustris*—Mississippi pine—Sea-coast of Carolina and Florida. Product: Boston turpentine; yields one-sixth of good oil; false elemi, resin for making soap, and the best tar for cordage.
"*Pinus strobus*—Weymouth pine—Virginia. Product: American turpentine; more fluid than the others, and yields more oil; is mixed with Boston turpentine.
"*Pinus cembra*—Siberian stone pine—European Alps. Product: A very fluid turpentine; its branches macerated in water, and distilled, yield the Carpathian balsam.

"Section II.—*Firs.*
"*Abies taxifolia*—Silver fir—European Alps. Product: Strasburgh turpentine; yields two resins, the one, deposited in blisters, remains clear and fragrant; the other, furnished by incision, gets turbid, and resembles pitch.
"*Abies balsamea*—Balm of Gilead—North America. Product: Spurious balsam of Gilead, deposited in blisters, preserves its limpidity, smell and strength. Balsam of Canada obtained by incision is less fragrant, less clear, and thicker.

"*False Firs.*
"*Abies picea*—North of Europe and Asia. Product: White pitch; a thick resin, at first clear, then turbid and soon hardens; very little oil.
"*Abies canadensis*—Hemlock spruce—North of America. Product, considered resinous, of which is made the North American pitch, which is tar boiled down to one-half.
"*Abies nigra*—Black spruce—North of America. Product: Black essence; constitutes more than two-thirds of the tar of Ohio, Lake Champlain, as far as Newfoundland.
"*Abies orientalis*—Levant spruce. Product: Spruce tears; resin exuding naturally from the extremities of the branches, remains clear.

"*Larches.*
"*Larix europœa*—Common larch—European Alps. Product: Venice and Briançon turpentine; occurs rather towards the centre of the tree, and sometimes in small reservoirs; the most employed in pharmacy; yields also Briançon manna; and also manna of Oremburgh, according to Pallas.
"*Larix cedrus*—Cedar of Lebanon—Syria,

Caucasus. Product: Cedar resin; yields also a saccharine substance, the cedar honey of the ancients, analogous to a Briançon manna; young seeds filled with a resinous acrid juice.

"*Pinus dammara*—Oval-leaved larch—Mountains of Amboyna. Product: White dammar; its oil evaporates very quickly, and there results a resin as hard as stone.

"*Dombeya excelsa*—Aracauria imbricata—Norfolk island pine. Product: Glutinous turpentine, of a milky whiteness; the body of the tree, according to some, contains none.

"*Thuya articulata*—North of Africa. Product: Sandarac, a dry resin; flows by incision, or, according to Desfontaines, naturally."

Dr Duncan's own remarks are valuable and well worthy of attention.

"All the tribe abound in every part with resinous juice, which possesses the same general qualities, but presents some varieties, according to the nature of the species and mode of preparation."

The turpentines obtained from some species are stimulant, diuretic, and cathartic. They are seldom given internally, but are occasionally prescribed in gleets, *fluor albus*, and in some varieties of asthma. The balsam of copaiba, which in its chemical constitution resembles the turpentines, has now superseded the real turpentines, that is to say, the produce of the pines, in all affections of the urinary organs.

The oil of turpentine is a medicine of a highly stimulating nature; in small doses it acts as a powerful diuretic, frequently causing strangury, with bloody urine. In large doses it acts as a violent purgative, and has been long used as a vermifuge. Dr Fenwick of Durham proposed its use in tape-worm, and it has been employed with the utmost success in that affection. Large doses seldom cause either strangury or hæmaturia. In combination with *Ol. Ricini*, it is one of the most efficacious purgatives with which we are acqainted. In cases of torpid action of the bowels, and in the latter stages of fever, where the powers of life are at a low ebb, enemata containing oil of turpentine are valuable stimuli. Dr Duncan says, that "in obstinate constipation it stands without a rival. In enteritis, peritonitis, colic, and certain inflammatory and spasmodic affections of the abdominal viscera, it acts almost as a specific. It is also efficacious in checking the hæmorrhage in dysentery; and Dr

Magee has used it with success in *hæmorrhœa petechialis*. Some habits cannot bear oil of turpentine. I have seen large doses produce temporary intoxication, and sometimes a kind of trance, lasting twenty-four hours, without, however, any subsequent bad effect. The largest dose I have known to have been given has been three ounces, and without injury." The oil of turpentine, whether taken internally or applied to the skin, communicates to the urine the smell of violets. Externally, it acts as a rubefacient, and produces excellent effects in chronic rheumatism, in indolent swellings, in paralysis of the extremities, and in spasmodic affections. It has also been applied to burns. Mixed with boiling water in equal proportions, and applied to the stomach and abdomen as hot as the patient can bear it, it frequently succeeds in putting a stop to the most obstinate vomiting. Applied in the same way to the extremities, it acts more rapidly, and in some cases more beneficially than sinapisms would do. To sloughing ulcers, and in gangrene, whether arising from frost-bite or from old age, turpentine dressings are most useful. Of the other products of the pine tribe, tar and pitch are both used in medicine. Tar water and the vapour of boiling tar have been recommended in phthisis, and pitch has been prescribed with the best results in ichthyosis.—See Dr Bateman on Cutaneous Diseases, and Dr Elliotson's Lectures on Clinical Medicine.

COMMON MALLOW

Malva sylvestris

Class and Order, Monadelphia Polyandria. Nat. Ord. Malvaceæ.
Gen. Char. *Styles* numerous; *Calix* double, exterior of three leaves; *Capsules* numerous, circularly arranged, one-seeded.

———————————

Root perennial, long, thick and fleshy; stems several, two to four feet high, much branched; flowers large, purplish red, growing three or four together from the axils of the leaf-stalks. The whole plant is mucilaginous, particularly the seeds and roots, and, from the abundance in which the species is found in most parts of Britain, may be advantageously substituted for the marsh-mallow, *Althœa officinalis*, which is comparatively of rare occurrence, their properties being identical.

Pl. 36.

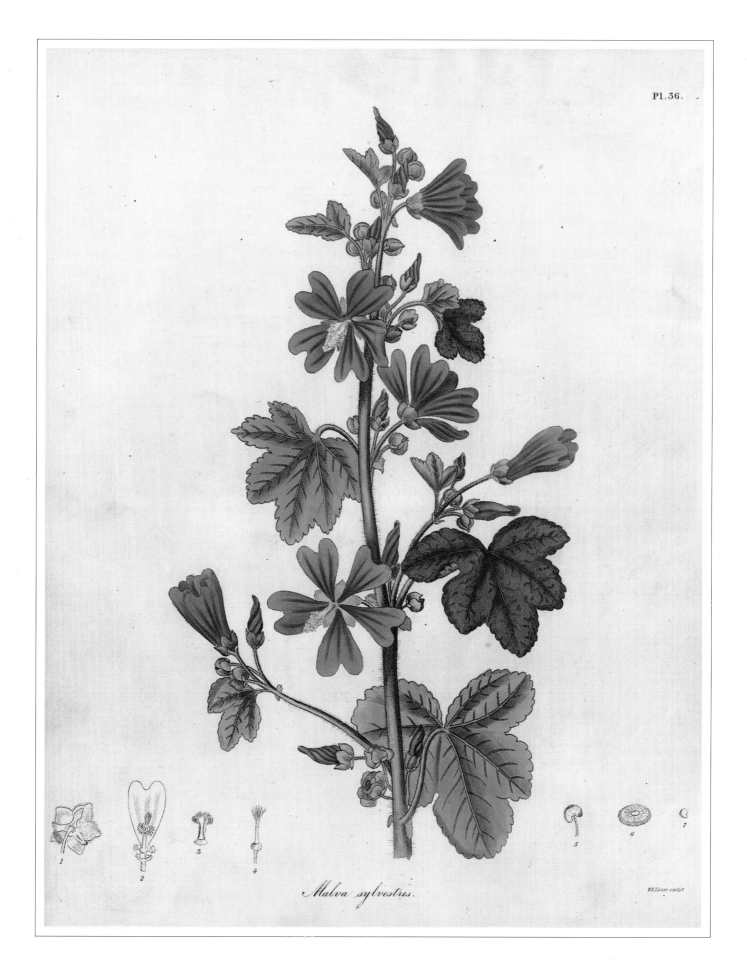

Malva sylvestris.

W.H.Lizars sculpt

COMMON MALLOW

The whole of this natural family abounds in mucilage, and, though of considerable extent, there is no individual known that is possessed of noxious qualities, being all nutritious, emollient, and mucilaginous. The common mallow is found on banks and in hedge-rows, and when in blossom, is particularly conspicuous from its large and handsome flowers, which are produced in great profusion from June to September. Seventy-five species are described in *Don's System of Gardening and Botany*.

From the quantity of mucilage which the common mallow contains it is frequently used as a demulcent. In the form of a decoction it is administered in chronic diarrhœas and in diseases of the bladder. In France, an infusion of the flowers is frequently prescribed in irritation of the bronchiæ and mucous membranes.

A decoction of the leaves and roots is used as an emollient glyster, and the leaves and roots themselves are made into poultices.

COMMON COTTON

Gossypium herbaceum

Class and Order, MONADELPHIA POLYANDRIA. NAT. ORD. MALVACEÆ.

Gen. Char. *Calix* double, cup-shaped, bluntly five-toothed, exterior three-leaved, leaflets connected at the base, cordate, jagged; *Stigmas* three or five; *Capsule* three or five-celled, many seeded; *Seeds* enveloped in cotton.

THE plants producing cotton, though not at present introduced into the British Pharmacopœias, merit particular notice, as furnishing a substance which has of late years been most advantageously employed in cases of severe burns and scalds. The most convenient preparation of this article is that known in domestic use by the term wadding.

Gossypium is thought to be derived from the Arabic word *Goz* or *Qoz*, which signifies any soft or silky substance, from which is derived the Latin name. The down or cotton is found almost filling the capsules, and closely investing the seeds. Seventeen species are described, but there is much to learn of this interesting genus. The *herbaceum* is the only species cultivated in Europe for economical purposes, particularly in the Levant, Malta, Sicily, and Naples; it is likewise grown in many parts of Asia. This species is sown in spring, and yields its crop in the following October. The *hirsutum* is grown in the West Indies, but the *Barbadense* is the species generally cultivated; it is sown in drills in the beginning of October; and rises six feet high, yielding two crops annually. In the East Indies the *arboreum*, which rises to a tree twelve feet high, is cultivated. A bland oil is extracted from the seeds of the *herbaceum*, which is used for culinary and domestic purposes.

The species which produces the cotton of which NANKEEN CLOTH is manufactured is supposed to be the *religiosum*; its cotton is at first of a deep buff, almost copper colour, which by washing and exposure finally assumes the tint usually known by the term nankeen. Pliny says that cotton was manufactured into garments for the Egyptian priests.

The filaments or threads of cotton are barbed, so as when in close contact to adhere firmly together. Manufacturers have taken advantage of this; and cotton manufactured into a variety of fabrics constitutes a large proportion of the clothing of most of the inhabitants of civilized countries. The British cotton factories are probably the most extensive in the world, and afford employment to an immense part of the population.

The seeds of the Bombax, or silk cotton tree, are surrounded by a substance called silk-cotton; the trees are among the largest of the countries they inhabit. The trunks of the *B. ceiba* in the West Indies are sometimes so large that they are hollowed and used as canoes, and are capable of carrying twenty-five tons or more.

An East India species, the *pentandrum*, rises to more than an hundred feet high, and produces a fruit the size of a swan's egg, which opens into five parts and is filled with a short dark-coloured silky cotton. In consequence of the threads or filaments being perfectly smooth, it is incapable of being manufactured into cloth, but in its raw state is equally efficacious when applied to recent burns or scalds.

MARSH-MALLOW

Althæa officinalis

Class and Order, MONADELPHIA POLYANDRIA. NAT. ORD. MALVACEÆ.

Gen. Char. *Styles* numerous; *Calix* double, exterior, of six to nine leaves; *Capsules* numerous, circularly arranged, one-seeded.

THE Marsh-Mallow is most abundant in marshes near the sea. It is clothed with a dense pubescence, which renders the leaves exquisitely soft; it attains two or three feet in height, and has large, showy, pale rose-coloured flowers, often tinged with blue. It is in great estimation on the continent of Europe, particularly in France, and its mucilage is formed into lozenges for pectoral complaints.

The *Althea officinalis* does not differ in its medicinal properties from the common mallow; it contains even more mucilage than that plant. A proximate vegetable principle was discovered in it by M. Bacon, and named by him *Altheine*. This has been examined by M. Plisson and various other continental chemists, and is now named *Asparagine*.

SENNA

Cassia

Class and Order, DECANDRIA MONOGYNIA. NAT. ORD. LEGUMINOSÆ.
Gen. Char. *Calix* five-leaved; *Petals* five, equal; *Stamens*, three superior sterile, three lower beaked; *Legume* membranaceous, two-valved.

THE uncertainty prevailing as to the plant producing what is called Senna, has tended greatly to the introduction of various kinds of *Cassia leaves, as those of the officinal species, as well as the leaves of a considerable variety of other plants.* Whether the leaves vary in form on the same plant, we are ignorant; but the figures given by foreign as well as English writers are by no means sufficiently determined to identify the species.

All the true Sennas have the portions of their leaves unequally divided. In some kinds the lower part of one side is reduced to little more than a line in breadth, whilst the other is from a quarter to half an inch in breadth. The Cassias form an extensive family, and are found in the warmer parts of both hemispheres.

That drug known under the name of East Indian senna is nearly free from adulteration; and as its properties appear identical with those of the Alexandrian, and the price being less, it probably will supersede it in general practice. Its size and shape readily identify it.

No drug in the Materia Medica is subject to more considerable and noxious adulterations than that known in the shops as Alexandrian senna,—an article imported from the Levant, and various parts of Greece and Turkey, where several species are indigenous. The old officinal name of *Cassia senna* is very properly discarded, the officinal senna being a compound of the leaves of a variety of species, which appear to possess similar properties, the principal of which are *C. lanceolata, C. obovata* and *C. obtusata*. These, when free from any other admixture, form the genuine Alexandrian senna; but it is rarely found in the drug market in this state.

The adulterations are exceedingly numerous, as the finest samples that can be procured in our drug warehouses evidently attest; but there is considerable obscurity as to the articles surreptitiously introduced, from their being mostly so broken down that entire leaves are not readily found. Of those with which we are best acquainted I have annexed correct figures. One of the most noxious is the *Coriaria myrtifolia*, a plant belonging to the natural family of *Coriariæ*, and possessing very poisonous properties. The leaves of this plant when entire may always be detected by their regular shape, and the peculiar arrangement of the veins; it is an adulteration much more common on the continent of Europe than in this country. With respect to the Argel, *Cynanchum oleæfolia*, Dr Christison suggests, "the adulteration is obviously not a fraud, but intended to form a specific mixture."

Another common but spurious leaf and seed-vessel, abounding in most of the Alexandrian and Tripolian sennas, belong to a species of *Tephrosia*. These will be immediately known, the leaves being of a regular form.

Of all the fictitious senna leaves, the least injurious, or, I may perhaps justly say, the most beneficial, are the leaves of the *Colutea arborescens*, the common bladder-senna. They possess cathartic properties, appear equally powerful, and are quite devoid of the nauseous taste and smell of the true drug; and, should a course of experiments now in progress confirm the present opinion, it may probably supersede the use of senna.

Senna is a useful and common purgative. It is usually given in the form of infusion, and is very certain in its operation; it is admissible in most diseases, and is only objectionable from its nauseous taste, and from occasionally giving rise to tormina. The first of these objections is got rid of by mixing the infusion with molasses, or, according to Dr Paris, by adding the infusion of Bohea tea, and mixing cream and sugar with the united infusions in the same way as with common tea. The second objection is also got rid of by adding some aromatic, such as ginger, or coriander seed. The syrup of senna, which is prepared with molasses, is an excellent medicine for children, as it is easily taken, and is mild in its operation. The leaves of the *C. acutifolia*, which are known in this country by the name of "East Indian senna," are the produce of Arabia Felix; they are much milder in their operation than the leaves of *C. lanceolata*, "Alexandrian senna," and seldom cause griping, and are coming into general use; they are very highly esteemed in India.

MARYLAND WORM-GRASS OR CAROLINA PINK

Spigelia marilandica

Class and Order, Pentandria Monogynia. Nat. Ord. Gentianæ.
Gen. Char. *Corolla* funnel-shaped; *Stigma* simple; *Capsule* two-celled, double.

The Spigelia is a naive of North America, possesses a perennial root, and is not of easy cultivation in England. I have succeeded with it in the open border, by planting it in a pot, in the bottom part of which was a quantity of fragments of pots to afford a ready drain of excessive moisture; the soil should be a sandy peat mixed with loam, and the pot should be plunged in the border. Stems about a foot high, four-sided, the leaves growing in opposite pairs; flowers terminal, growing from one side of the stem and placed on short footstalks, the blossoms open in succession, commencing from the bottom, and rarely more than two or three are expanded at one time. This plant is used as a vermifuge in North America. Another species, common in the West Indies, *S. anthelmia*, is extensively used for the same purpose.

The *Spigelia marylandica* is very seldom employed medicinally. The root and leaves are both active. They have a bitter nauseous taste, and

are sometimes used in intermittents. Dr Duncan mentions, that an emetic is generally prescribed before the Spigelia is given; he also mentions, that Dr Barton recommends an infusion of the root "in the insidious remitting fever of children, which often lays the foundation of hydrocephalus."

PURGING CATHARTOCARPUS

Cathartocarpus fistula

Class and Order, Decandria Monogynia. Nat. Ord. Leguminosæ.
Gen. Char. *Calix* of five leaves, deciduous; *Corolla* regular, of five petals; lower filaments bowed; *Pod* long, round, woody, many-celled; *Cells* filled with pulp.

This species forms a tree of from thirty to forty feet in height, and produces its leaves of five pairs of leaflets, of a delicate green, oblong, and pointed. Flowers large, showy, and fragrant; pods about an inch in diameter, and from one to two feet in length, which at first are green, but as they advance to maturity, become of a deep-brown; the seeds are enclosed in separate parti-

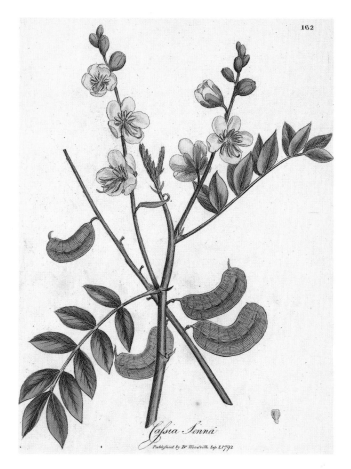

Cassia Senna
Published by Dr Woodville Sep. 1.1792

SENNA

tions, or cells, which are, when ripe, filled with a black pulpy substance, possessing considerable cathartic powers, from which circumstance the plant has obtained its present generic appellation.

A native of the East Indies and Africa; has been cultivated in Great Britain since 1731.

SCAMMONY

Convolvulus scammonia

Class and Order, Pentandria Monogynia. Nat. Ord. Convolvulaceæ.
Gen. Char. *Corolla* campanulate; *Capsule* two-celled, two-seeded; *Stigma* two-cleft.

Root long, tapering, fleshy, throwing numerous tender stems, which, like all the climbing species of Convolvuli, entwine themselves round any stems or twigs they come in contact with. They extend to a great length, sometimes to nearly twenty feet; flowers pale sulphur colour, growing out from all parts of the stems. The drug scammony is procured from the roots, which are cut off obliquely at the crown,—some vessel being introduced so as to receive the juice that runs from the wounded part; when this is hardened it forms the scammony of the shops, but it is frequently adulterated by being mixed with sand and other impurities.

Scammony is a native of the Levant, Turkey, Syria, Persia, and Cochin-China.

As a drug it is a drastic purgative and vermifuge. It ought to be prescribed in combination with some demulcent, when given without the addition of some other purgative, as it is apt to cause tormina. The action of scammony is very similar to that of jalap. The best comes from Aleppo, but even this is occasionally adulterated with flour, sand, or earth; when pure, it is in light spongy masses, of a dark ash colour, of a disagreeable heavy smell. A very inferior kind is brought from Smyrna.

JALAP

Ipomœa jalapa

Class and Order, Pentandria Monogynia. Nat. Ord. Convolvulaceæ.
Gen. Char. *Corolla* funnel-shaped; *Capsule* three-celled; *Stigma* capitate.

The plant producing jalap is a native of Mexico. It is an elegant twining plant, the root large and spindle-shaped, from which arise numerous slender stems, as in the *Calystegia sepium*. The flowers are sometimes of a dark crimson, at others of a pale rose-colour; large, of only one day's continuance, but as they are produced in considerable abundance, the plants are rarely without blossom during the season. It is presumed that the specific name of the plant as well as the drug jalap, is derived from Xalapa, near Mexico, where the plant is found wild, and from which the roots are imported. One hundred and nine species are mentioned in Hortus Britannicus.

Jalap is a safe and effective purgative. In moderate doses it acts without causing tormina, but in an over-dose it excites hypercatharsis and violent pain, and sometimes produces dangerous symptoms; Dr Christison, speaking of its poisonous qualities says, "this every one ought to know, as severe and even dangerous effects have followed its use in the hands of the practical joker." In combination with calomel, jalap forms one of the most valuable purgative formulæ, especially in local inflammation,—in ophthalmia for example.

Orfila quotes M. Felix Cadet de Gassicourt's Inaugural Dissertation on Jalap at full length, from which it appears that jalap proves fatal when rubbed into the skin for a length of time, or when placed in contact with the pleura, or when given in a large dose, but not when injected into a vein. There seems from the above statements considerable uncertainty as to what the active principle of jalap really is. The subject is worthy of further investigation.

COMMON DOG-ROSE

Rosa canina

Class and Order, Icosandria Pentagynia. Nat. Ord. Rosaceæ.
Gen. Char. *Calix* urn-shaped, fleshy, contracted at the orifice, terminating in five segments; *Petals* five; *Pericarps* numerous, bristly, attached to the inside of the calix.

The dog-rose varies in depth of colour from almost pure white to a deep red, also with double or semi-double flowers, and the varieties are interminable. Upwards of three hundred

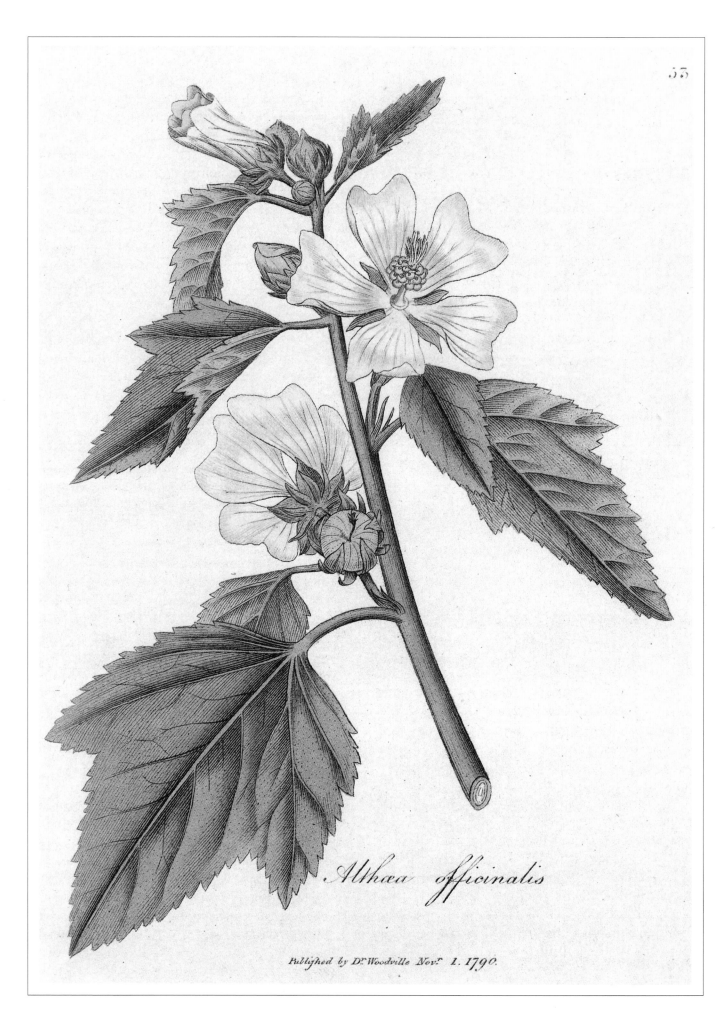

Althæa officinalis

Published by Dr. Woodville Novr. 1. 1790.

MARSH MALLOW

varieties of the Scotch rose, *Rosa spinossissima* are to be found in some nurseries. Of the present species, Professor Hooker enumerates five varieties, to which may be referred the following species of different authors, *canina, sarmentacea, glaucophylla, sarculosa, venosa, dumetorum, Forsteri, collina, campestris*; but it is of no material consequence to the practitioner from which of the varieties he obtains the fruit, which is the only officinal part. The fruit or hep has an agreeable acid taste, and is ripe about the month of September, but in many kinds they remain on the bushes during the winter; yet if deferred to be gathered until the frost commences, they lose much of their acidity.

The petals of the dog-rose are not used medicinally. A conserve is prepared from the fruit, which is sometimes prescribed as a demulcent. The utmost care is necessary in preparing this conserve, as the small sharp hairs which surround the seeds create great irritation in the throat and fauces.

HUNDRED-LEAVED ROSE

Rosa centifolia

Class and Order, Natural Order, and Generic Character, see *R. canina.*

THE present species, a native of the south of Europe, was formerly the most commonly cultivated of garden roses, but since the rage for varieties, it has sunk into comparative neglect: it forms a bush from three to six feet high, and produces a profusion of flowers, whose fragrance is not surpassed by any of the more showy kinds. This fragrance, which is so esteemed in the open air, soon becomes oppressive in a confined room, and even life has been endangered by persons being confined in rooms with a quantity of the flowers. From experiments by Drs Priestley and Ingenhousz, this effect was considered to arise from *mephitic* gas, exhaled by this and other odoriferous flowers, which spontaneously diffuse their odours. Nearly one hundred varieties of this species are to be met with in Britain's gardens, and so great is the demand for varieties of roses, that in certain London nurseries upwards of fourteen hundred named sorts are cultivated.

The *Rosa centifolia* is chiefly valued for the fragrance of its flowers; it is or ought to be used in the distillation of rose-water, but this is rarely done, the rose-water which is usually met with being made by adding an alcoholic solution of the essential oil to distilled water. The essential oil, otto, attar, or uttir, is prepared in Turkey, Persia, and other eastern countries, and is very highly esteemed as a perfume. Various species are used in its preparation, but the *centifolia, sempervivens, damasena,* and *moschata* yield the greatest quantity, and the highest flavoured oil. Berzelius gives the following account of the distillation of the attar: Alternate layers of rose leaves and the seeds of a species of *Digitalis* are placed in contact; the seeds contain a large quantity of fixed oil, which absorbs the essential oil of the leaves; fresh portions of leaves are added to the same seeds, which, when fully impregnated, are pressed, and the oil which exudes is separated from the watery juice by means of fine cotton. This oil, which consists of the fixed oil of the seeds and volatile oil of roses, is distilled, and the oil which passes over is the pure attar.

It varies in colour, but is usually of a lemon yellow. Dr Duncan mentions that Colonel Polier "had attar of a fine emerald green, of a bright yellow, and of a reddish hue in the same year, from the same ground, and by the same process, from roses collected on different days.

The petals of the *R. centifolia* are occasionally given as laxatives, and a syrup prepared from them is frequently administered to children. In India the leaves of the *moschata* are occasionally prescribed.

OFFICINAL ROSE

Rosa gallica

Class and Order, Natural Order and Generic Character, see *R. canina.*

THIS, like the preceding species, is a native of the south of Europe, but has long been an inhabitant of Britain's gardens. It is of more humble growth than the *centifolia*, with deeper coloured flowers, the petals of which, though large, are not nearly so numerous, nor does it possess the fragrance so much admired in that species. Loudon mentions nearly two hundred varieties of this species; all the kinds are of easy cultivation, growing readily from layers, cuttings, or seeds, from the latter new varieties are raised;

they all prefer a pure air, but some kinds bear the smoke of large towns uninjured, whilst others are almost immediately destroyed in the same situations.

The petals of the *Rosa gallica* are valued for their fine colour and for their astringency; but they possess but little fragrance. An infusion prepared from them, and acidulated with sulphuric acid, is an excellent gargle in relation of the throat, and is a very good vehicle for nauseous drugs. A confection is prepared by grinding the fresh petals with sugar, and is much used for giving consistence to pills and boluses. It is sometimes prescribed as an astringent.

COMMON RUE

Ruta graveolens

Class and Order, Decandria Monogynia. Nat. Ord. Rutaceæ.
Gen. Char. *Calix* five-parted; *Petals* five, concave; *Receptacle* with ten nectariferous glands; *Capsule* lobed.

Rue is a native of the south of Europe, but bears the cold of our climate without injury. It is a low perennial shrub, with glaucous foliage, and greenish-yellow flowers, and is too well known to require description. It was formerly used in the service of the Roman Catholic church for sprinkling the holy-water among the congregation, from whence it derived its appellation of Herb of Grace.

Every part of the Rue has a strong, aromatic, and rather disagreeable, odour, and a bitter, aromatic, and somewhat acrid, taste. It is held in considerable repute on the European Continent. It is stimulant, emmenagogue, and diuretic. Richard says that it ought to be given with great caution, as it is apt to cause uterine hemorrhage, inflammation of the uterus, and, under certain circumstances, abortion. It is used as a vermifuge principally by the country people, with whom it is a favourite plant. It contains about a four-hundredth part of its weight of an essential oil, to which it owes its taste, smell, and medicinal properties. This oil is of a greenish or yellow-brown colour, which deepens by age. When exposed to cold it freezes, and regularly-formed crystals may be observed. Rue was held in great estimation by the ancients, both as a culinary and medicinal herb.

LAVENDER

Lavandula spica

Class and Order, Didynamia Gymnospermia. Nat. Ord. Labiatæ.
Gen. Char. *Calix* ovate, somewhat obtuse, supported by a bractea; *Corolla* resupinate; *Stamens* included within the tube.

This species is a native of the south of Europe, but is extensively cultivated in many parts of Britain. It forms a low shrubby plant, from two to four feet in height, is of ready growth, and thrives well in soils that are too sterile for most other plants. Stems shrubby, the older ones covered with a loose dry bark; leaves numerous, linear, entire, hairy beneath, with the edges revolute; flowers of a light delicate purplish blue, growing in interrupted whorls.

Lavender is fragrant, aromatic, stimulant, and antispasmodic; it is useful in hysteria and the nervous complaints of females; but it is chiefly valuable as a perfume. Immense quantities are grown for the use of the perfumer, who manufactures from the flowers an essential oil, which is the base of the majority of perfumes. The *Lavandula vera*, or narrow-leaved lavender, yields the most fragrant oil; the *L. spica*, which is called the officinal species, is not so often used in the preparation of the oil, as it is much less fragrant.

Oil of lavender, according to Proust, deposits about one-fourth of its weight of stearoptine, which he considers identical with camphor, and from which he proposes camphor should be procured for medicinal purposes.

COMMON BALM

Melissa officinalis

Class and Order, Didynamia Gymnospermia. Nat. Ord. Labiatæ.
Gen. Char. *Calix* dry, flattish above, with the upper lip somewhat fastigiate; *Upper lip* of the corolla flat; lower crenate; *Anthers* cross-wise.

Root perennial, fibrous; stems erect, from one to two feet or more high, quadrangular, smooth, branching from the bottom; leaves heart-shaped, serrated, of a lively green, standing on long foot-stalks; flowers white, with pale red spots, growing in whorls, which only half sur-

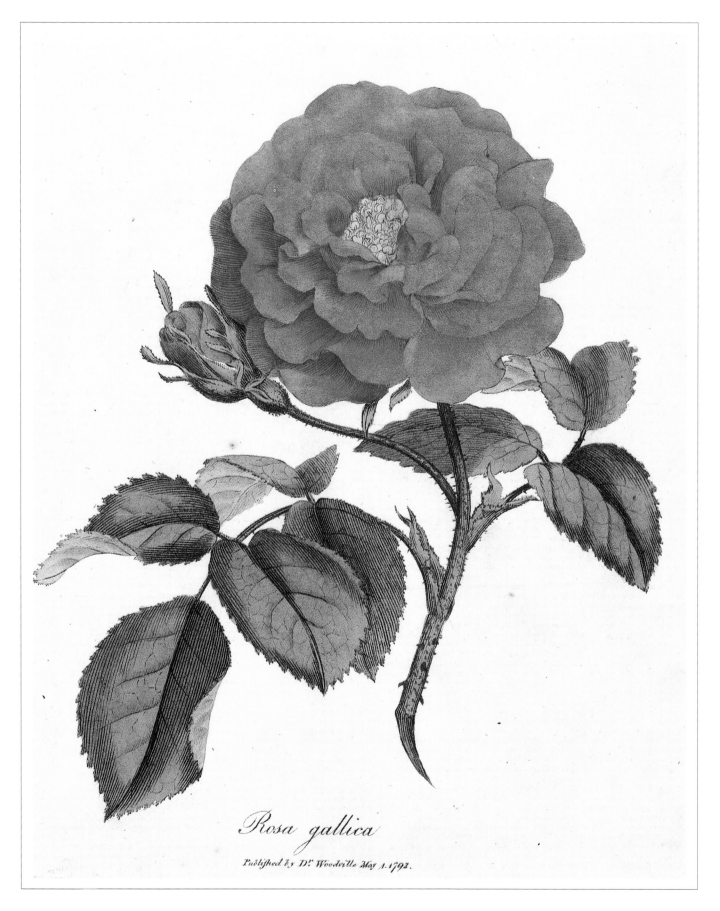

Rosa gallica

Published by Dr Woodville May 1. 1792.

OFFICIAL ROSE

round the stalks. The whole plant has an agreeable scent, and was formerly held in much estimation.

Balm is a native of the south of Europe, but thrives well in Northern Europe.

The common balm is occasionally prescribed in the form of infusion as a gentle tonic. It contains a very small quantity of volatile oil, having an odour resembling that of bergamotte and mint. Balm-tea is a common popular remedy in many complaints, especially in diseases of the bladder.

COMMON COW-AGE OR COW-ITCH

Stizolobium pruriens

Class and Order, Diadelphia Decandria. Nat. Ord. Leguminosæ.
Gen. Char. *Calix* campanulate, two-lipped, upper lip entire, erect, lower trifid, with the middle segment longest; *Vexillum* ascending, wings axe-shaped, lunate at the base, the length of the *carina*; *Anthers* hairy; *Legume* uneven, one-celled with partitions; *Seeds* round, with a crested hilum.

The pods of this species, as well as *S. urens*, are thickly covered with a dense prickly tomentum, which is the officinal part of the plant, and is used as a vermifuge. Cow-age is native of the East and West Indies, where it grows in great luxuriance, climbing to the summits of the tallest trees; it is a perennial plant, with ternate leaves, and handsome purple flowers. Its pods are imported from the West Indies, and the hairs are scraped off with a knife for use; they are so sharp as to penetrate the skin, when they occasion an intolerable itching; a similar inconvenience is occasioned by the hairs of several species of caterpillar.

An infusion of the root of the Stizolobium is used by the native practitioners of India in Cholera. The pods of this plant are covered with stiff brown hairs; these are scraped off and mixed with thick syrup or honey, and prescribed as anthelmintic. This remedy is frequently used in the West Indies, and in general with success, the worms that are voided are said to be always found transfixed with some of the hairs. Much irritation follows the insertion of one of these hairs or setæ into the hand or arm.

COMMON QUINCE

Cydonia vulgaris

Class and Order, Icosandria Pentagynia. Nat. Ord. Pomaceæ.
Gen. Char. *Calix* five-parted, with leafy divisions; apple closed, many-seeded; *Testa* mucilaginous.

The Quince is a low tree, with numerous branches; leaves ovate, entire, downy beneath; it is a native of many parts of Europe, and, though long cultivated for medicinal purposes, it possesses no qualities that are not more advantageously obtained from other substances. The seeds are the only officinal part, yielding an impure mucilage with boiling water.

The quince has a somewhat austere, acid taste, and is seldom eaten till quite decayed; conserves of various sorts are prepared from it. The seeds contain a large quantity of mucilage, which is occasionally employed as a substitute for Gum-Arabic, but as it is incompatible with acids, and very readily enters into a state of fermentation, it has never been much used.

WHITE HOREHOUND

Marrubium vulgare

Class and Order, Didynamia Gymnospermia. Nat. Ord. Labiatæ.
Gen. Char. *Calix* with ten ribs, and five or ten spreading teeth; the throat hairy; *Corolla* with the tube exserted; *Upper lip* straight, linear, cloven; lower one three-lobed, middle lobe the largest, emarginate.

Root perennial, fibrous; stalks upright, one foot, to one and a-half high; leaves deeply serrated; flowers white, in crowded whorls; stems and leaves thickly coated with a white pubescence, which gives the whole plant a hoary appearance.

Common horehound is a stimulant tonic expectorant; its taste is bitter, and slightly acrid, and its odour strong and unpleasant. It is principally used as an expectorant, and is occasionally of service, though it does not deserve the encomia which have been at different periods lavished on it. Many empirical preparations bearing the name of preparations of horehound are sold; of these perhaps the safest is the tablet, as it is not so likely to contain foreign matters, being com-

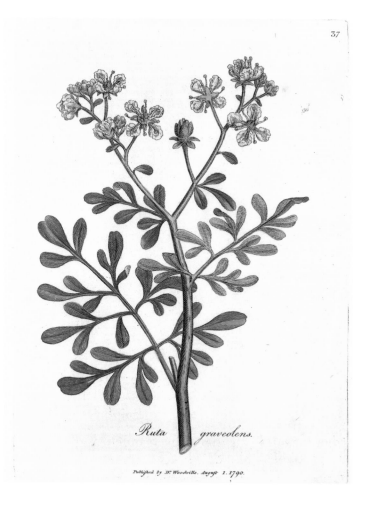

Ruta graveolens.

Published by D.r Woodville, August 1.1790.

37

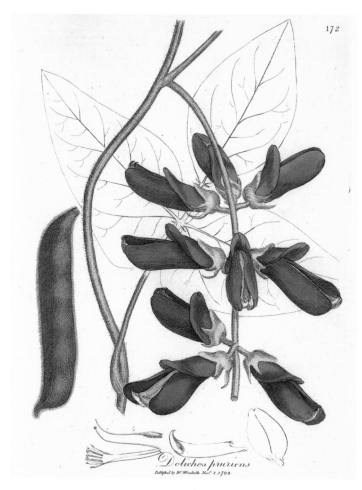

Dolichos pruriens

Published by D.r Woodville Nov.r 1.1792.

172

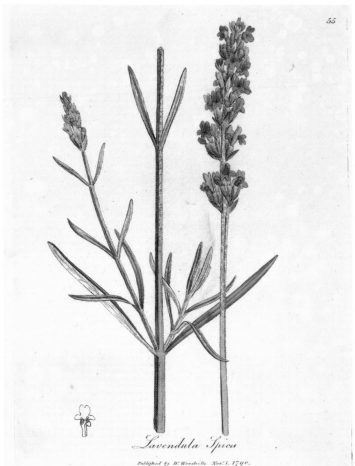

Lavendula Spica

Published by D.r Woodville Nov.r 1.1790.

55

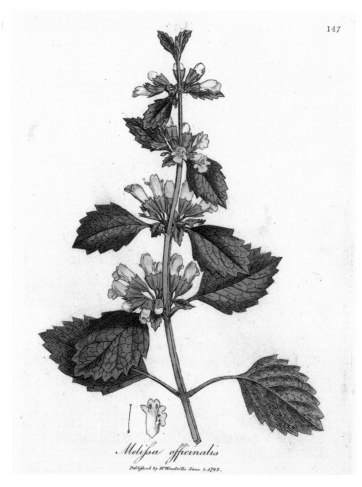

Melissa officinalis

Published by D.r Woodville June 1.1792.

147

TOP LEFT: COMMON RUE, TOP RIGHT: COMMON COW-AGE OR COW-ITCH, BOTTOM
LEFT: LAVENDER, BOTTOM RIGHT: COMMON BALM

monly prepared by the confectioner. As to the liquid preparations, they are dangerous, from containing a quantity of spirit, which is not the best addition to an expectorant. In some varieties of asthma, and in chronic catarrh, horehound has been occasionally useful.

It contains essential oil, on which its odour and stimulant qualities depend; bitter extractive; gallic acid and tannin.

EGYPTIAN THORN OR GUM-ARABIC TREE

Acacia vera

Class and Order, Nat. Ord. and Generic Character, see
A. Catechu.

THOUGH the present plant is supposed to yield the drug known in the markets as Gum-Arabic, little doubt exists but that the same substance is produced by a considerable variety of Acacias, as well as other trees; and various kinds of stone fruit, as the plum, almond, and cherry, produce a substance resembling the finest Gum-Arabic. I have often used pieces gathered from cherry trees, which answered all the purposes of the true kind, for mixing with water colours. As to the identity of the tree which produces the Gum-Arabic of commerce, there is no satisfactory information which would induce us to attribute the produce to any particular species.

The *Acacia vera* is a low tree of stunted growth, and unsightly appearance, the stem is covered with a smooth grey bark, the branches have a purplish tinge; the leaves grow alternately, and are composed of two pairs, each of which is composed of eight or ten pairs of leaflets. It is a native of sandy places in Barbary and Morocco. The best kind is that found in pure colourless or rather frothy-like tears, and exudes spontaneously from the tree.

The Gum-Arabic of commerce is obtained from several species of Acacia. The best is said to be the produce of the *Acacia vera*. Dr Duncan says, "there are two kinds of gum found in the shops of England, and often sold promiscuously, but distinguished in common by the names of Gum-Arabic and East India gum. Gum-Arabic consists of roundish transparent tears, colourless, or of a yellowish colour, shining fracture, without smell or taste, and almost perfectly soluble in water. The pieces which are most transparent and have least colour are reckoned the best. They are sometimes selected from the Gum-Arabic in sorts, and sold for about double the price, under the title of picked gum. The East India gum is darker coloured than Gum-Arabic, and is not so readily soluble in water. Again, "about the middle of November, that is after the rainy season, which begins early in July, a gummy juice exudes spontaneously from the trunk and principal branches. In about fifteen days it thickens in the furrow down which it runs, either in a vermicular shape, or more commonly assuming the form of round or oval tears about the size of a pigeon's egg, of different colours, as they belong to the white or red gum tree. About the middle of December, the Moors encamp on the borders of the forest, and the harvest lasts six weeks. The gum is packed into very large sacks of tanned leather, and is brought on camels and bullocks to certain ports, where it is sold to the merchants. Besides Gum-Arabic, all the species produce an astringent juice, analogous to catechu, and used for similar purposes. Gum-Arabic is used in medicine in all cases where there is a deficiency of the mucous lining of the intestines, in cases of bronchitis, in phthisis, both as a demulcent and for nutriment; in acrid poisoning, to defend the coats of the stomach. Externally it is applied as a mechanical styptic, as an injection in gonorrhœa and in ulceration or irritation of the rectum. I have found strong mucilage very useful in severe diarrhœa, and have given about half a pound of gum in this way for two or three days consecutively.

MARJORAM

Origanum vulgare

Class and Order, DIDYNAMIA GYMNOSPERMIA. NAT. ORD. LABIATÆ.
Gen. Char. *Calix* various; *Corolla* with the upper lip erect, nearly plane, lower one patent, trifid.

A HARDY perennial of common occurrence in dry hilly situations; stems very erect, much branched at the summit; flowers purple; calix and bracteas frequently of the same hue; in the present species the branches of flowers are very diffuse, but some of the foreign kinds have the heads four-sided, resembling catkins imbricated with bracteas; leaves entire, or slightly indented on the edges. Though retained in the Pharmacopœias, it has no peculiar properties different from the other nearly allied genera in this truly natural family.

The *Origanum vulgare* is considered tonic, emmenagogue, and stimulant. Its odour is similar to thyme, and it yields a considerable portion of essential oil, which possesses its virtue in a concentrated form.

KNOTTED MARJORAM

Origanum majorana

Class and Order, Nat. Ord. Generic Character, see *O. vulgare.*

A native of Portugal and the warmer parts of Europe, and much in request for culinary purposes; it requires the shelter of a frame in this country, and is usually treated as a tender annual, though commonly of longer duration. It produces its flowers in dense clusters or knots, from whence it acquires its common appellation of Knotted Marjoram.

The *Origanum majorana* is officinal, but is very rarely used; it enters into the composition of vegetable cephalic snuffs, and is fully more agreeable than the *vulgare*. It is much used as a pot-herb.

COMMON MULBERRY

Morus nigra

Class and Order, Monœcia Tetrandria. Nat. Ord. Artocarpeæ.
Gen. Char. Male; *Calix* four-parted; *Corolla* wanting. Female; *Calix* four-leaved; *Corolla* wanting; *Styles* two; *Calyx* berried; *Seed* one.

The common or black mulberry has been cultivated in Britain since 1548. It is a native of Italy, but bears the cold of Britain's climate without injury. It is a tree of very slow growth, and of great longevity; many of those in the neighbourhood of London are suppposed to have been planted during the reign of James the First, and are now in full vigour, or scarcely attained their full size. Contrary to other fruits, this becomes larger and finer on the oldest trees, that produced by young trees being comparatively tasteless. The leaves of this and other species are used as food for silk-worms; for which purpose considerable numbers have been of late years planted in the south of Ireland, for the purpose of introducing the growth of silk into this country; the species usually employed is the *M. alba*, or white mulberry, the fruit of which is of a pale-green, almost white, and is of a less acid taste than the common species. The fruit should be used as soon as gathered, as it becomes mouldy in a few hours after being taken from the tree.

The fruit of the mulberry is sweet, subacid, and mucilaginous. It is seldom used in medicine, but is in much request for the table. The bark of the tree is acrid and bitter, and has been suggested as a remedy in *tænia*. The leaves are considered the best food for silk-worms.

ICELAND MOSS

Cetraria islandica

Class and Order, Cryptogamia Algæ. Nat. Ord. Lichenes.
Gen. Char. *Thallus* foliaceous, cartilagineo-membranaceous, ascending and spreading, lobed and laciniated, on each side smooth and naked; *Apothecia* orbicular, obliquely adnate, with the margin of the *thallus*, the lower portion being free, (not united with the *thallus*;) the *Disk* coloured, plano-concave, with a border formed of the *thallus* and inflexed.

An abundant species, principally confined to northern and alpine regions. It is found in various parts of Scotland, but does not produce fructification except on some of the more elevated mountains. Most of that used in England is imported from Norway or Iceland, and it is to the natives of those countries an equivalent to bread. It has a bitter unpleasant taste, which is in great part removed by maceration in cold water. It is principally used as an article of diet. It is nutritive and easy of digestion. Other species of this family likewise possess nutritive properties; the *Tripe de Roche,* (*Gyrophora*) common to the Arctic regions, was the principal food on which Sir Thomas Franklin and his adventurous associates were compelled to subsist for a considerable time; and it is more than probable that a number of our native lichens would form a wholesome, if not a very palatable, food, as many of them contain large quantities of starch.

Iceland moss has been highly extolled as a cure for phthisis, but its curative power has not been as yet very apparent. It is nutritious, and is a very good substitute for arrowroot, or any other mucilaginous article of diet. Before using it, it ought to be steeped in water, to which a little potass has been added, that the bitter taste which it has made be destroyed. It may be afterwards boiled in milk or cocoa.

DYER'S ROCCELLA OR ARCHILL

Roccella tinctoria

Class and Order, Cryptogamia Algæ. Nat. Ord. Lichenes.
Gen. Char. *Thallus* coriaceo-cartilaginous, rounded or plane, branched or laciniated; *Apothecia* orbicular, adnate with the thallus; the *Disk* coloured, plano-convex, with a *border*, at length thickened and elevated, formed of the *thallus*, and covering a sublentiform, black, compact, purulent powder, concealed within the substance of the thallus.

Archill is found on the maritime rocks in the south and west of England, but does not appear to be known in any part of Britain. That used in dyeing is principally procured from the Canary Islands, and is imported in immense quantities; it is usually in small tufts, and often mixed with other species of sea-weed.

RED SAUNDERS TREE

Pterocarpus santalinus

Class and Order, Diadelphia Decandria. Nat. Ord. Leguminosæ.
Gen. Char. *Calix* five-toothed; *Legume* falcate, foliaceous, varicose, indehiscent, encompassed by a wing; *Seeds* few or solitary.

The tree producing the saunders wood is lofty, with alternate branches, and a bark resembling the common alder. The wood is imported in billets. It is very heavy, sinking in water; of a bright garnet-red colour, which deepens on exposure to the air, and aromatic smell; is exceedingly hard, fine-grained, and susceptible of a high polish.

The wood of the *Pterocarpus santalinus* is only useful or interesting as a dye. It is seldom or never used in medicine for its medicinal virtues. It contains a peculiar colouring matter, insoluble in water, soluble in alcohol and some of the weaker acids, to which the name of *Santaline*

has been given. It is obtained by acting upon the wood with ammonia, and by precipitating the alkaline solution with muriatic acid. The *Santaline* when thus obtained is in the form of a brownish-red colour. Its alcoholic solution precipitates the metallic salts, and with some forms beautiful pigments.

MASTICH-TREE

Pistacia lentiscus

Class and Order, Diœcia Pentandria. Nat. Ord. Anacardiaceæ.
Gen. Char. Male: *Calix* five-cleft; *Corolla* wanting. Female: *Calix* three-cleft; *Corolla* wanting; *Styles* five; *Drupe* one-seeded.

This species is a native of the south of Europe. It is a low tree or shrub, seldom exceeding ten or twelve feet in height, much branched at the summit; the leaves are pinnate, composed of six or eight pairs of leaflets, placed on winged foot-stalks; flowers growing three or four spikes together, from the axilla of the leaves, and sometimes are terminal; as in the former species, the flowers are inconspicuous.

Mastich is obtained from incisions made in the bark, from whence it exudes, and is received on cloths, to keep it free from impurities; when hardened, it is of a light yellow colour, brittle and hard, and usually is imported in small round fragments.

Mastich is the concrete resinous juice of the *Pistacia lentiscus*; it is much used by the Turks and other eastern nations as a masticatory (hence its name;) but in Europe it is chiefly used for making varnishes and cements.

CYPRESS TURPENTINE-TREE

Pistacia terebinthus

Class and Order, Natural Order and Generic Character, see *P. lentiscus.*

A native of Greece, the south of Europe, and north of Africa, but thrives well in cooler climates. The tree seldom exceeds twenty feet in height, has pinnate deciduous leaves, and produces its spikes of inconspicuous flowers at the end of the wood formed the year preceding. On being wounded, the turpentine exudes, and

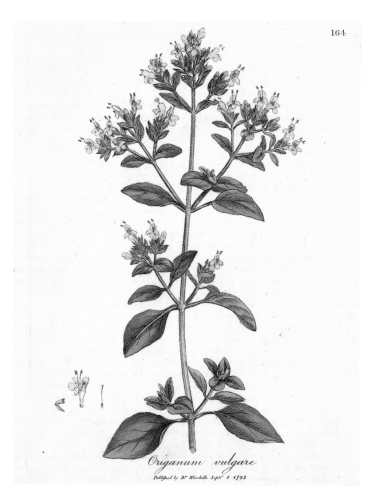

Pistacia Lentiscus

Published by Dr Woodville July 1.1792.

152

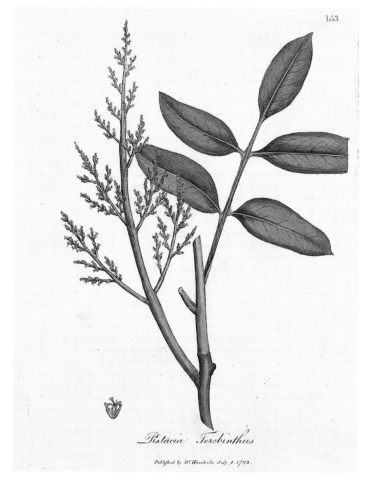

Origanum vulgare

Published by Dr Woodville Sept. 1 1792.

164

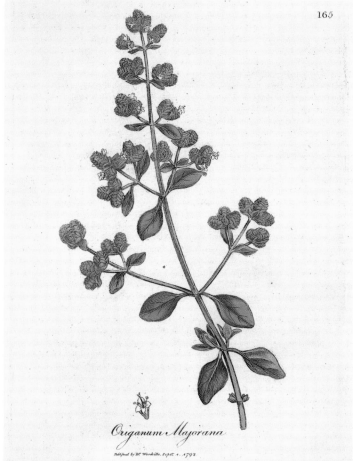

Origanum Majorana

Published by Dr Woodville Sept. 1. 1792.

165

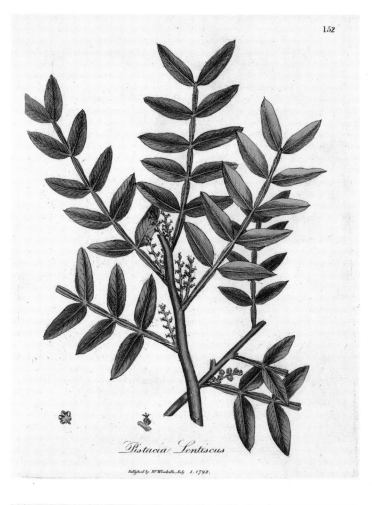

Pistacia Terebinthus

Published by Dr Woodville July 1.1792.

153

TOP LEFT: MASTICH TREE, TOP RIGHT: MARJORAM, BOTTOM LEFT: KNOTTED
MARJORAM, BOTTOM RIGHT: CYPRESS TURPENTINE-TREE

103

when hardened, forms the drug cypress turpentine.

The Chian or cypress turpentine is the produce of the *Pistacia terebinthus*. It does not differ from the other turpentines, but it is more fragrant, much higher priced, and frequently adulterated.

EUROPEAN ORNUS OR MANNA-TREE

Ornus europœa

Class and Order, Diandria Monogynia. Nat. Ord. Oleaceæ.
Gen. Char. *Calix* four-parted; *Corolla* of four petals; *Fruit* a winged *Samara* of two cells.

This plant with one or two others were separated from the genus Fraxinus by Persoon, and form that of Ornus. They differ from the true ash, in having a calix and corolla, of which that tribe are destitute.

The present species is common in Greece and the south of Europe; it is a low tree, in aspect resembling the common ash, but has smaller foliage, which are on long grooved foot-stalks, placed opposite, composed of several leaflets, and a terminal one; the flowers are in loose panicles, white, and situated at the extremities of the branches; capsules pendulous, of a similar form to those of the ash, vulgarly called keys.

Manna is the concrete juice of the tree, in the trunk of which an incision is made, and something introduced to convey the juice to the air, upon exposure to which it hardens. It is produced by a variety of other trees, but this is cultivated for the express purpose. The finest kinds are in the form of small tubes, occasioned by pieces of straw or stick being introduced into the parts from whence the juice exudes, which, flowing upon these, hardens, and is more valuable than what is in mass, from its containing less impurities.

The concrete juice of the *Ornus europœa* is called Manna. It exudes spontaneously from the tree, and is also obtained by making incisions. The best is imported from Sicily and Calabria, and is produced without incisions having been previously made. It is frequently adulterated by the admixture of honey and sugar; and an artificial manna is prepared by mixing honey and sugar with a small quantity of scammony. It

is a gentle and pleasant laxative, but its action is so mild that it is generally combined with some more powerful cathartic, such as senna or rhubarb. A variety of sugar, to which the name of *Mannite* has been given, was discovered by Proust in the manna obtained from the *Ornus*. The same variety of sugar has been found in many other plants, such as onions, beet, celery, asparagus, the larch, &c.

TAMARIND-TREE

Tamarindus indica

Class and Order, Monodelphia Triandria. Nat. Ord. Leguminosæ.
Gen. Char. *Petals* three, ascending, three fertile filaments longer than the others; *Legumen* one to three-celled, pulpy within.

The tamarind forms a large spreading tree. Its leaves are abruptly pinnate, composed of sixteen or eighteen pairs of sessile leaflets; calix pale straw-coloured, deciduous; flowers full yellow, elegantly veined with deep red. These are succeeded by pods of a roundish compressed form, from three to six or eight inches in length: seeds bright mahogany-coloured, flat, angular, and shining, lodged in the pulpy lining of the pods. This, which is the only known species, is common to both Indies, and also Arabia and Egypt. The officinal preparation is merely the pulp preserved by the addition of syrup. That obtained from the West Indies is to be preferred.

The fruit of the tamarind preserved with sugar is useful in febrile diseases as a gentle laxative. Hot water poured on it acquires a sweet, subacid, agreeable taste, and is a very palatable drink; it allays thirst, and is cooling in its effects.

COMMON FIG-TREE

Ficus carica

Class and Order, Polygamia Diœcia. Nat. Ord. Artocarpeæ.
Gen. Char. Common receptacle turbinate, closely, fleshy.
Female: *Calix* five-parted; *Corolla* wanting; *Ovary* one; *Seed* one.
Male: *Calix* three-parted; *Corolla* wanting; *Stamens* three.

The species are either trees or shrubs abounding in a milky juice. In temperate climates such as Britain, the fig rarely ripens its fruit in the open

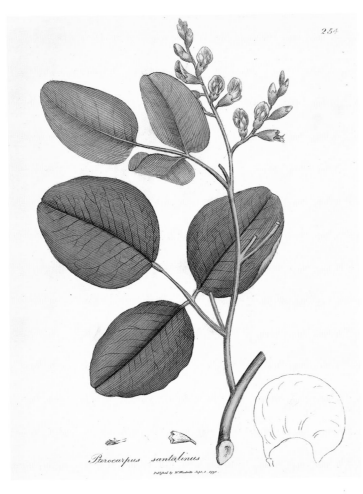

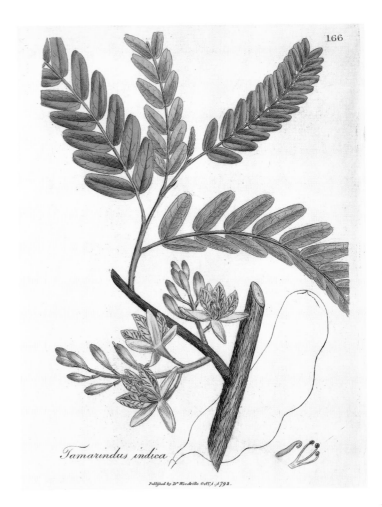

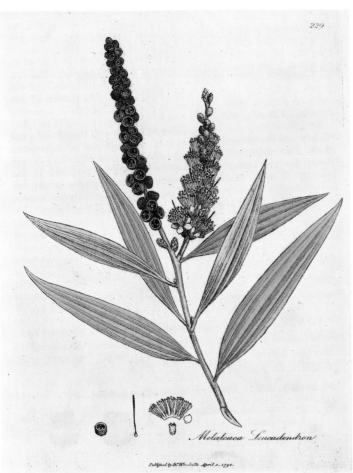

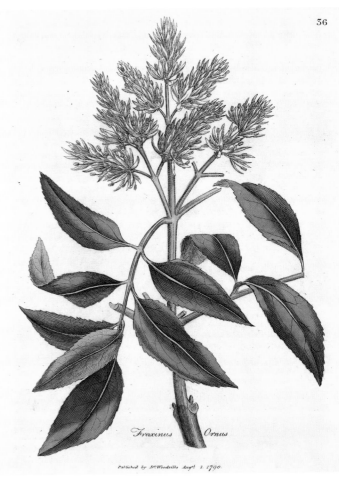

TOP LEFT: RED SAUNDERS TREE, TOP RIGHT: TAMARIND-TREE, BOTTOM LEFT:
CAJAPUTI TREE, BOTTOM RIGHT: EUROPEAN ORNUS OR MANNA TREE

ground, though it grows luxuriantly and produces quantities of fruit, which fall off without coming to perfection. The ripe fruit is exceedingly sweet and luscious, but is not held in much esteem in this country; the dried fruit is imported from Turkey and the Levant, particularly the Faroe Isles. This is an extensive genus, comprehending seventy-four known species, besides varieties, the whole of which are natives of warm climates.

In the natural family to which this genus belongs are found the bread-fruit, *Artocarpus incisa*, the jack, and the mulberry, and, as remarked by Professor Lindley, "are a curious instance of wholesome or harmless plants in an order containing the most deadly poison in the world,—the *Upas* of Java." He adds, "the juice, however, of even those which have wholesome fruit is acrid and suspicious; and in a species of fig, *Ficus toxicaria*, is absolutely venomous." *F. indica* is a tree of immense size, spreading very wide, the branches ash-coloured, and throwing down roots into the soil. One is mentioned by Marsden growing near Memgee, twenty miles west of Patna in Bengal, which was in diameter 370 feet, the circumference of the shadow at noon was 1116 feet, and there were fifty or sixty stems; it was called the Priest's tree, and was held in great veneration by the Gentoos; it is known in India as the Banyan Tree. *F. elastica*, with some other plants, produce the well-known substance, India-rubber.

Figs are more properly articles of food than of materia medica. They consist almost entirely of sugar and mucilage, and are very good demulcents. They act as gentle laxatives, and are useful in habitual consitpation. A roasted fig is a popular remedy in gum bile, and it seems to promote suppuration with a great rapidity.

HEMLOCK

Conium maculatum

Class and Order, Pentandria Digynia. Nat. Ord. Umbelliferæ.

Gen. Char. *Calix* obsolete; *Petals* obcordate, inflexed at the points; *Fruit* laterally compressed, ovate; *Carpels* with five prominent, waved, or crenated equal *ridges*, of which the lateral ones are marginal; *Interstices* with many *striæ*, without *vittæ*; *Seed* with a narrow groove in front; *Universal involucre* of *few leaves*; partial of *three leaves on one side*.

Root biennial, fusiform, whitish; stems from two to five feet high, much branched at the top, channelled, and spotted with red purple; root leaves large, much divided; cauline ones smaller, finer cut. This plant closely resembles several others of Britain's native umbelliferæ, but is readily distinguished by its spotted, smooth, and shining stems, also by its powerfully fetid odour when bruised. Its root is large, often from a foot to eighteen inches in length, and from an inch to an inch and a-half in diameter, and has much the appearance of a parsnep. When boiled, the roots appear destitute of any deleterious quality, and I have repeatedly eaten them; their taste resembles that of parsnep, but is less sweet; to me their taste has nothing peculiar to recommend them, but at the same time it is not unpleasant; nor do they produce any injurious effects.

The same method should be adopted in drying the hemlock for medicinal purposes, as mentioned in describing the Digitalis.

Hemlock was well known to the ancients, but had fallen into disuse; it was re-introduced by Dr Stoerk in the middle of the eighteenth century, and was said by him to be successful in the removal of scirrhous tumours; it alleviates the pain in open cancer, and can be employed both internally and externally. In its effects it resembles opium more than any of the other umbelliferous narcotics; and in constitutions where that drug is inadmissible, it is a valuable substitute. The leaves are the officinal part, and are more active than the root, which is by some authors said to be nearly inert, but this opinion must have arisen from less active plants having been mistaken for Conium or from the root having been dug up at an improper time. In man, the effects from an overdose are similar to what an overdose of opium causes. Dr Christison quotes from Corvisart's Journal the following cases of poisoning with this plant: "M.——, a French army surgeon, has described a fatal case of poisoning with hemlock, which closely resembled poisoning with opium. The subject of it, a soldier, had partaken, along with several comrades, of a soup containing hemlock leaves, and appeared to them to drop asleep not long after, while they were conversing. In the course of an hour and a-half, they became alarmed on being all taken ill with giddiness and headach, and the surgeon of the regiment was sent for. He found the soldier, who had fallen asleep, in a state of insensibility, from which, however, he could be roused for a few moments. His countenance was bloated, the pulse only 30, and the extremities cold. The insensibility became rapidly deeper and deeper till he died, three hours after taking the soup. His companions recovered." The extreme fluidity of the blood is a remarkable circumstance in cases of poisoning with Conium. In the case above quoted, "on opening the head a quantity of blood flowed out, which twice filled an ordinary chamber-pot." Dr Christison found the blood remarkably fluid in a case which he examined; and he mentions, that Dr Coindet of Geneva found that a small quantity of the infusion of Conium prevented blood from coagulating even when removed from the body.

The powdered leaves are the most certain of the preparations of Conium, but they require to be carefully prepared and preserved, and to be prescribed with the utmost caution. The extract is a very convenient preparation, but its strength is uncertain, unless when prepared in vacuo from plants collected at the proper season, which is when the plant is flowering. In hooping-cough and phthisis, Conium has been found useful, and in rheumatism complicated with paralysis, it has succeeded in effecting several cures. In conjunction with calomel, it has proved beneficial in various inflammatory diseases where opium could not with propriety have been given.

CAJAPUTI TREE

Melaleuca leucadendron

Class and Order, POLYADELPHIA POLYANDRIA. NAT. ORD. MYRTACEÆ.
Gen. Char. *Stamens* long, in five bundles, opposite the petals; *Anthers* incumbent; *Capsule* three-celled, many-seeded, connate, and included in the thickened tube of the calix, which is grown to the branch.

IT IS probable that more than one species of Melaleuca yield the oil known in commerce as Cajeput oil. The species above described is generally esteemed as the officinal plant; it is a native of the East Indies and islands in the Indian ocean; it forms an upright tree of moderate size, with longish pendant branches and leaves; the bark is whitish ash-colour; spikes of flowers are terminal, with a leaf bud at the extremity, which before the flowers are all developed expands into a leafy twig, by which flowers appear to grow from the centre of the branch.

Cajeput oil is obtained from the leaves of the Melaleuca by distillation; it is of a bright-green colour, and a pungent aromatic camphorous taste; its green colour was supposed to arise from the presence of copper, as it is brought to Europe in copper flasks; but Mr Brande could not detect a trace of the metal. As an external application, Cajeput oil is useful in chronic rheumatism, in weakness of the joints arising from oil dislocations or sprains, and in indolent tumours. It is used internally like the other essential oils, and is said to be more powerfully anti-spasmodic. In *Cholera spasmodica* it was at first considered a specific, but it afterwards fell into complete neglect.

BALSAM OF GILEAD-TREE

Amyris gileadensis

Class and Order, OCTANDRIA MONOGYNIA. NAT. ORD. AMYRIDEÆ.
Gen. Char. *Calix* four-toothed; *Petals* four, oblong, spreading; *Stigma* capitate; *Berry* drupaceous, one-seeded.

THE tree which yields the Balsam of Gilead is an evergreen, twelve feet or more in height, with a thick stunted stem; leaves growing in threes; branches purplish, somewhat striated; flowers ternate, white, succeeded by a purplish brown berry, containing a smooth nut, flattened on one side and furrowed. This species is supposed to produce the celebrated Balm of Gilead, which is among the most ancient of medicinal drugs. It is a native of Arabia, but the trees are scarce, and the produce of balsam so very trifling that its price is exhorbitant, and renders it always subject to adulteration.

Balm of Gilead is hardly ever procured in a state of purity in this country; as it does not possess any virtues which the other balsams do not, its scarcity is not of much importance. It has been used from the earliest periods; it is spoken of in Scripture; and is still in high repute in the East. It is much more aromatic than any of the other balsams, and in this lies its only superiority.

Pl. 37.

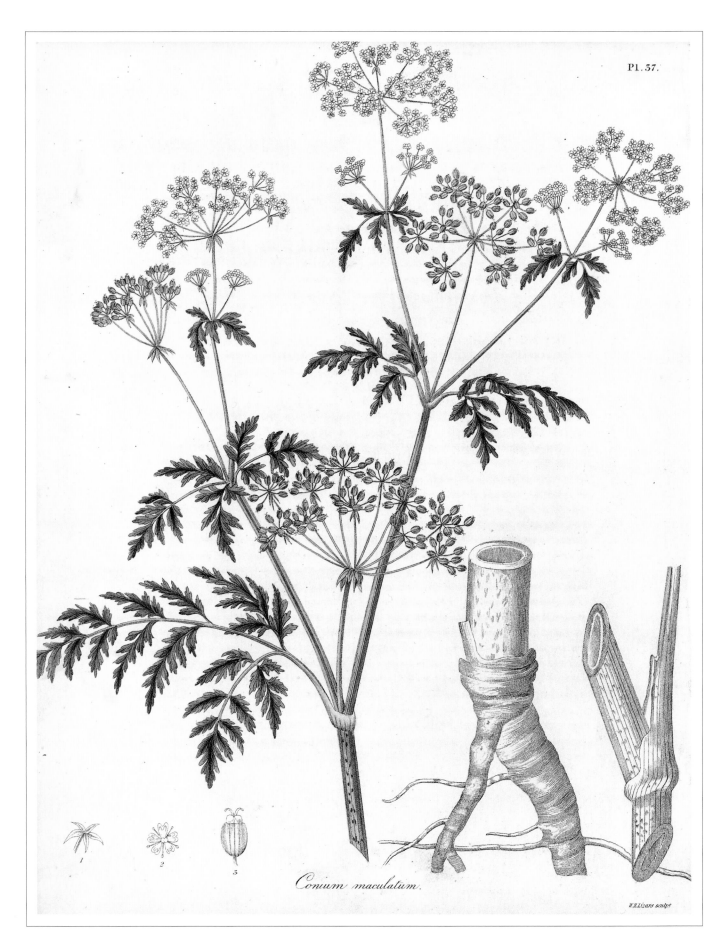

Conium maculatum.

W.H.Lizars sculp.

HEMLOCK; FIG.1, CALIX; FIG.2, FLOWER; FIG.3, SEED MAGNIFIED

BALSAM OF PERU-TREE

Myroxylon peruiferum

Class and Order, Decandria Monogynia. Nat. Ord. Leguminosæ.
Gen. Char. *Calix* cup-shaped, five-toothed; *Petals* five, the superior one larger than the others; *Legume* with one seed.

THE tree which produces the Balsams of Peru and Tolu is described as growing in Mexico and Peru; is of moderate size; the stem and branches covered with a coarse heavy bark, of a pale straw colour within, and filled with a fragrant resin that pervades every part of the tree.

"The balsam of quinquino (or Peru) is procured by incision at the beginning of spring, when the showers are gentle, frequent and short; it is collected in bottles, when it keeps liquid some years, in which state it is called white liquid balsam. But when the Indians deposit this liquid in mats or calabashes, which is commonly done in Carthagena, and in the mountains of Tolu, after some time it condenses, and hardens into resin, and is then denominated dry white balsam, or balsam of Tolu, by which name it is known in the druggist's shops."

Balsam of Tolu has a fragrant aromatic smell, and a warm agreeable taste; it acts as an expectorant, and is very often added to pectoral mixtures to cover the taste of less agreeable remedies. It contains volatile oil, but in such small quantity that it cannot be obtained in an uncombined state by distillation. Dr Duncan proposes that the syrup of Tolu should be prepared from the distilled water, instead of the tincture. Like the other balsams, it is composed of resin, benzoic acid, and, as already stated, volatile oil.

OFFICIAL STORAX-TREE

Styrax officinale

Class and Order, Decandria Monogynia. Nat. Ord. Styraceæ.
Gen. Char. *Calix* inferior; *Corolla* funnel-shaped, *Drupe* two-seeded.

THIS species is a native of Italy, and forms a low tree, with slender branches; leaves ovate, entire, hoary beneath; flowers white, growing in clusters from the sides, and terminating the young branches; fruit a juiceless globular drupe, containing two or three angular nuts. The drug storax exudes from incisions made in the bark.

The resinous concrete juice of the *Styrax officinale* is sold by the apothecaries, chiefly for the purposes of fumigation; it is used in the service of the Catholic church, and its perfume while burning is very agreeable. Storax contains benzoic acid, and an essential oil which cannot be separated by distillation. It is usually imported in bladders, and is frequently adulterated with benzoin, balsam of Peru, and saw-dust; it is very rarely employed in medicine.

BENZOIN STORAX OR BENJAMIN-TREE

Styrax benzoin

Class and Order, Nat. Ord. and Generic Character, see *S. officinalis*.

A native of Sumatra, forming a large tree, with long entire alternate leaves; flowers in straggling clusters, unilateral, of a dull white colour. The official preparation is obtained from the trees by incision in the bark, and the exudation allowed to harden by exposure to the air; it is then removed with a knife; it is imported in large masses; that which is the whitest, free from impurities, and breaking readily in the hand, is to be preferred; it is commonly mixed with chips, parings of the tree, and other extraneous substances.

Benzoin occurs in masses of an amygdaloid form, of a pale brownish red colour, streaked with whiter and darker portions; it was formerly used as an expectorant, but has now fallen into disuse. It is a good deal employed as a fumigatory, and enters into the composition of Pastilles. The smell while burning slowly and without flame is very agreeable, but from the quantity of benzoic acid which is formed, it causes considerable irritation in the nose, eyes, and larynx, if allowed to accumulate in a confined apartment.

The balsams all contain benzoic acid, and the usual definition of a balsam is, resin combined with benzoic acid and volatile oil. The Tonka (or *Tonquin*) bean also contains benzoic acid.

SEVILLE ORANGE

Citrus aurantium

Class and Order, Polyadelphia Polyandria. Nat. Ord. Myrtaceæ.
Gen. Char. *Calix* five-parted; *Petals* five, oblong; *Stamens* twenty, the filaments variously divided; *Berry* nine-celled.

ORANGES are imported from Spain and Portugal, and are extensively cultivated in Italy and the islands in the Mediterranean. Cultivated in the conservatory, they form low trees of a handsome form, with bright shining foliage, and are seldom to be seen without abundance of flowers and young fruit. These, to be brought to perfection, require the same attention as the peach or nectarine.

The trees, which rarely exceed eight or ten feet in height with us, are much branched, and frequently furnished with spines on the younger branches; leaves evergreen, of a deep shining colour, placed alternately, elliptical, with winged foot-stalks; flowers large, fragrant, fleshy, growing from the smaller branches; stamens small, about twenty; fruit a large pulpy globular berry, divided into nine compartments or cells, each of which contains from two to four seeds.

There are two varieties of this species, the sweet or China orange, and the bitter or Seville orange. The rind is used for the purpose of candying by the confectioner, and enters largely into the composition of most tonic mixtures. In its ripe state it is one of the most grateful and valuable of fruits; and, like other fruit trees that have been long under cultivation, is subject to considerable variation in the colour, form, and flavour of its fruit. Some foreign authors mention nearly 100 sorts of orange, but the specific differences are so obscurely pointed out that it is probable the larger part are mere seminal varieties. Loudon describes fourteen species of the genus.

The pulp of the orange contains a sweet subacid juice, which is grateful and cooling, and which is often prescribed in febrile and inflammatory diseases. The rind contains a fragrant essential oil, possessing stimulant and carminative properties, and a bitter principle, which is powerfully tonic. The flowers yield an essential oil, which is highly valued as a perfume, and which at one time was extolled as a cure for epilepsy and other convulsive diseases.

The distilled water of the flowers possesses calmative virtues, and is sometimes used instead of opium and its preparations. The acidity of the orange depends on the citric acid which it contains. The rind of the bitter orange is preserved by the confectioner in various forms. When boiled with sugar and dried, it is sold under the name of candied orange peel; when formed into a sort of jelly it is called *Marmalade*, and is in this state used for imparting flavour to various dishes, and as a preserve for the tea or breakfast-table. Orange peel, when simply dried, is an excellent tonic, and enters into the composition of many of our officinal bitters. Lebreton discovered a crystalline bitter principle in the unripe fruit, to which he gave the name of *Hesperidine*.

LEMON

Citrus limonum

Class and Order, Nat. Ord. and Generic Character, see *C. Aurantium.*

THE lemon greatly resembles the orange-tree, but has larger leaves, the foot-stalks of which are slightly winged; flowers white, or often with a faint blush of red; fruit oblong, pale-yellow, with a nipple-like apex. This elegant tree, in favourable situations, will bear the severity of British winters in the open air, but rarely ripens its fruit there, unless protected from the cold.

The lime greatly resembles the lemon, but is smaller in all its parts; the fruit when perfectly ripe has a sweetish pulp, but in its unripe state is more acid than the lemon. It rarely acquires more than six or eight feet in height, with occasionally thorns on its branches; the fruit is about an inch and a-half in diameter, nearly round, with similar protuberances as the lemon; it is smooth, of a greenish yellow-colour, and has a very fragrant rind.

The juice of the lemon is more acid than that of the orange, and is much more frequently employed in medicine. In union with the carbonate of potass or soda, it is commonly prescribed as a cooling saline effervescent in febrile diseases. The rind contains a large proportion of fragrant volatile oil, which is used as a perfume, and for giving the lemon flavour to various articles, such as lemonade, barley sugar, &c.

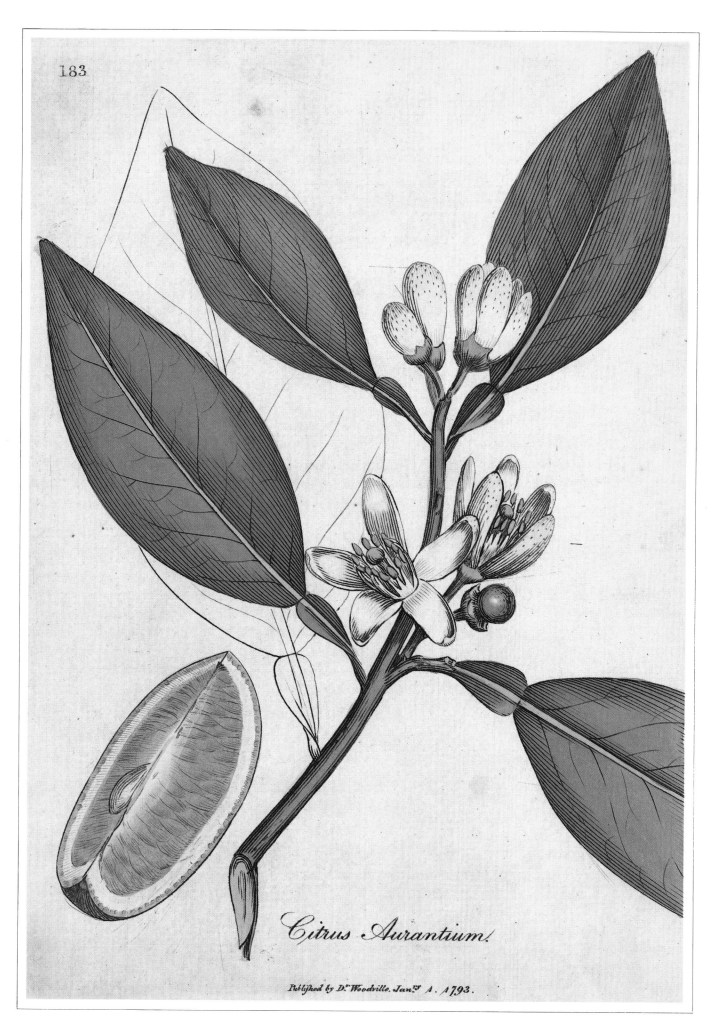

Citrus Aurantium.

Published by Dr Woodville. Jan.^{ry} 1. 1793.

SEVILLE ORANGE

ROUGH PARSNEP OR OPOPO-NAX

Pastinaca opoponax

Class and Order, Pentandria Digynia. Nat. Ord. Umbelliferæ.
Gen. Char. *Calix* nearly obsolete; *Petals* roundish, entire, involute with a sharp point; *Fruit* much compressed dorsally, with a broad flat border; *Carpels* with very slender *ridges*, the three intermediate ones equidistant, the two lateral ones remote, contiguous to the border; *Interstices* with single evident *vittæ*; *Seeds* flat. Universal and partial involucres of few leaves.

A hardy plant, which bears the rigour of winter in Northern Europe; it is a native of the south of Europe, the Levant, and neighbouring shores; it has a thick fusiform root, two or three feet long; the stems rise to six or seven feet high, and three or four inches in diameter; leaves large, rough on both sides; flowers in large umbels of a yellow colour.

The drug is obtained by wounding the root, from whence the juice issues and concretes; the finest sorts are in tears, that in mass is always loaded with impurities.

Opoponax is rarely used; it possesses emmenagogue and antispasmodic virtues; but so many medicines of a similar class are already in use, that it is not likely to become a favourite remedy.

STAVESACRE

Delphinium staphisagria

Class and Order, Polyandria Trigynia. Nat. Ord. Ranunculaceæ.
Gen. Char. *Calix* coloured, deciduous, irregular, upper leaflet protruded at the base into a spur; *Petals* four, two upper ones with appendages included within the spur.

A very ornamental plant; but, being a native of Italy and the warmer parts of Europe, does not succeed so well in the open ground as most others of the genus; it is an annual plant with showy flowers, growing from a foot to eighteen inches high; root-leaves large, palmated, gradually becoming smaller as they ascend the stem; stalks covered with dense hairs; flowers of a deep blue purple, redder at the edges, and deeper at the base; seeds rough, and black, angular.

Stavesacre seeds are acrid, nauseous, and bitter; they are rarely used internally, though they possess anthelmintic virtues of a very high order. They are most commonly applied externally when made into an ointment with axunge, for the purpose of destroying pediculi and other insects on the scalp and other parts. They owe their activity to a vegetable alkaloid, which was discovered in France by MM. Lassaigne and Fenuelle, and by Brandes in Germany at the same time. It is extremely poisonous.

SARSAPARILLA

Smilax sarsaparilla

Class and Order, Diœcia Hexandria. Nat. Ord. Smilaceæ.
Gen. Char. Male; *Calix* six-leaved; *Corolla* wanting. Female; *Calix* five-leaved; *Corolla* wanting; *Styles* three; *Berry* three-celled; *Seeds* one to three.

All the species of this genus are said to possess similar medical properties to the present one; the larger number of them are natives of America; our present plant is common in Virginia and several parts of South America. The drug which is imported as Lisbon Sarsaparilla comes from the Brazils, and is the most valuable; two or three other sorts are found in the drug market, besides some spurious kinds, as the root of the *Aralia nudicaulis*, *Carax arenaria*, and *C. hirta*, the two latter are called German Sarsaparilla, and are sometimes used as substitutes for the tree drug. In all the species of Smilax the pith or centre of the roots is white and ligenous, and all those kinds in which this is wanting may safely be rejected as spurious.

Root branched and fibrous, growing to the length of three or four feet, rather thicker than a goose-quill, externally brown, internally white; stems shrubby, long, slender and climbing, slightly angular, beset with strong scattered awl-shaped hooked spines; leaves ovate, with a short terminal point; flowers unisexual, inconspicuous; berry of a red-colour, the size of a currant, containing but one perfect seed. Loudon enumerates forty-one species.

Sarsaparilla was introduced by the Spaniards in the year 1563, for the cure of *Lues venerea*, and it is an example of the influence of fashion on medicines. When first introduced it was

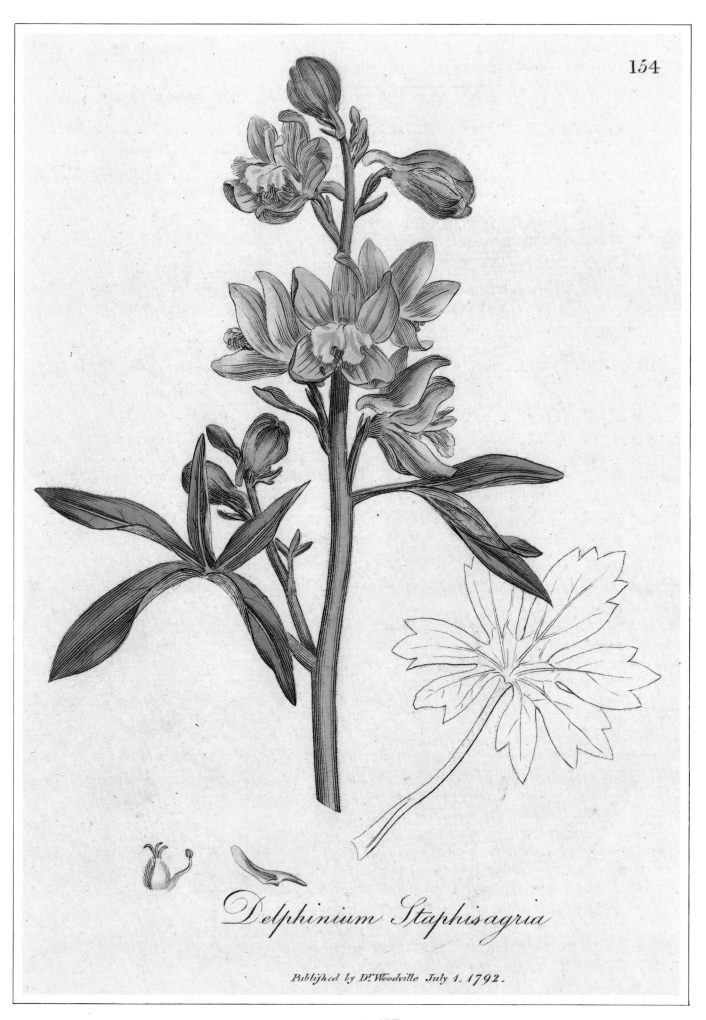

Delphinium Staphisagria

Published by Dr. Woodville July 1. 1792.

STAVESACRE

much praised, and came into extensive use. It then was entirely neglected, but has been revived of late years. Many practitioners trust entirely to sarsaparilla for the cure of primary syphilis, and have entirely discarded mercury; but it is in the sequelæ of syphilis that its good effects are most manifest. It seems to act as an alternative, for in many cases of general bad health unconnected with syphilis, or any other formed disease, the exhibition of sarsaparilla has effected a cure. According to Pallotta, the infusion of sarsaparilla when digested for some time with hydrate of lime yields a salifiable base (*Paragline*,) which is soluble in boiling alcohol, and which is deposited on cooling in the form of a white powder of a disagreeable bitter taste. It unites with and neutralizes the acids, and when taken into the stomach it causes nausea.

UMBEL-FLOWERED WINTER-GREEN

Pyrola umbellata

Class and Order, Decandria Monogynia. Nat. Ord. Pyrolaceæ.
Gen. Char. *Calix* five-cleft; *Petals* five, often connected at the base; *Anthers* opening with two pores; *Capsule* superior, five-celled; *Seeds* numerous, invested with a long arillus.

This beautiful species is dispersed over North America and the northern parts of Europe and Asia. Its flowers somewhat resemble those of *P. rotundifolia*, (a native species,) but are more showy. Root perennial, creeping; stems angular, erect, or slightly procumbent, four to six inches high; leaves in irregular whorls, lanceolate, deeply serrated, smooth, of a deep shining green; flowers in umbels of five or six, of a pale cream-colour, with the tips of the petals bright red; stamens ten, of a full purple-colour, which beautifully contrast with the delicate petals.

The *Pyrola umbellata* is much esteemed in America where the extract is used as a mild mucilaginous bitter in many diseases, particularly in nephritic and urinary affections, and the leaves are applied as external remedies in indolent ulcers, and even in cancer. As the extract is prepared in America, numerous adulterations are practised, and the extract must be considered an uncertain preparation.

RED BEAR-BERRY

Arbutus uva-ursi

Class and Order, Decandria Monogynia. Nat. Ord. Ericeæ.
Gen. Char. *Calix* deeply five-cleft; *Corolla* ovate, pellucid at the base; *Berry* superior, five-celled, many-seeded.

A native of the northern parts of England and Scotland, as well as of North America, and many parts of Europe; it is a dwarf procumbent shrub, with long trailing stems; leaves rigid, entire, edges revolute; flowers in small crowded terminal racemes, of a delicate rose-colour; fruit small, red, austere and mealy. It grows in dry heathy spots, and among rocks as a considerable elevation.

The leaves of the Arbutus have been much recommended as tonics in diseases of the kidneys and bladder. They are frequently employed in America. Their taste is bitter and somewhat astringent.

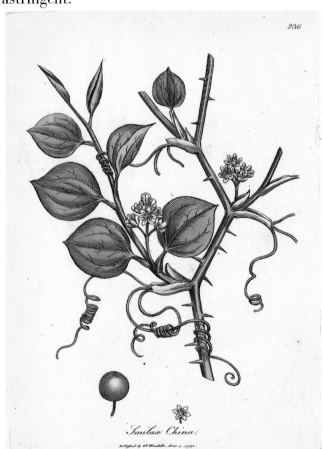

Smilax China.

SARSAPARILLA

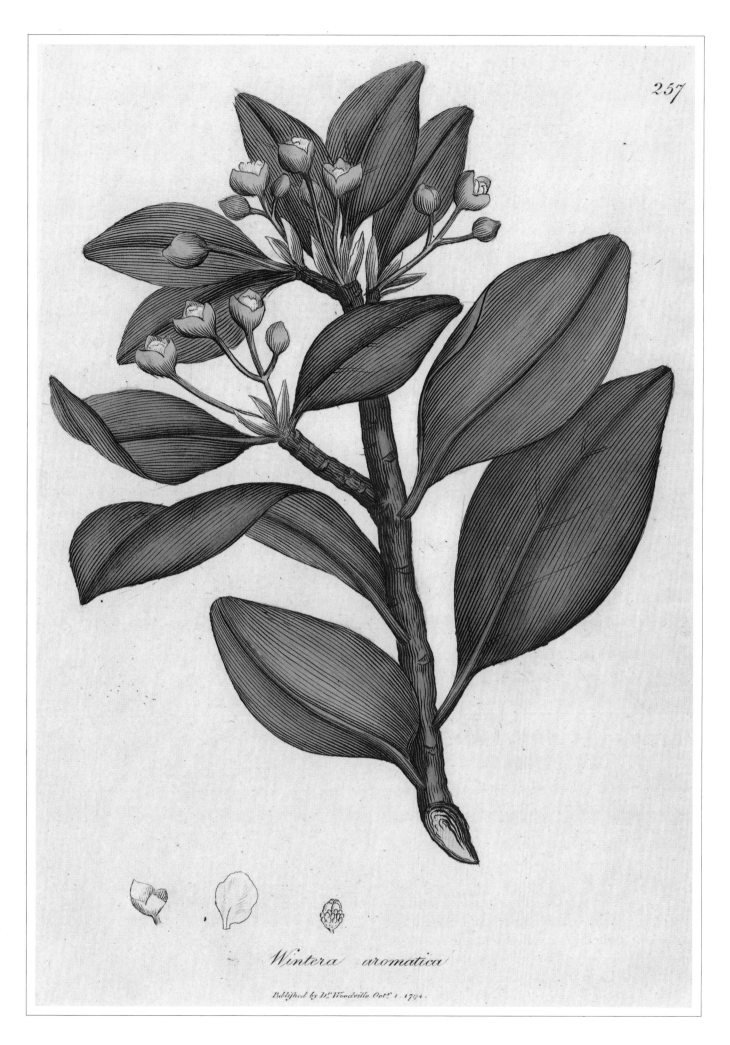

Wintera aromatica

Published by Dr. Woodville Octr. 1. 1794.

UMBEL-FLOWERED WINTER GREEN

VIRGINIAN SNAKE-ROOT OR BIRTH-WORT

Aristolochia serpentaria

Class and Order, Gynandria Hexandria. Nat. Ord. Aristolochiæ.
Gen. Char. *Perianth* superior, single, tubular, often swelling at the base; the *Mouth* on one side, dilated, one-lipped; *Stigma* with six lobes; *Capsule* inferior, with six cells.

A low perennial plant, a native of North America. Root-stock thick, fleshy; fibres numerous, slender; stems weak, slender, straggling, jointed, at each joint making an angular deviation, so that the stems are zigzag; leaves cordate; flowers dull-purple. Numerous species of this genus are used medicinally in different countries; formerly the *A. clematitis* was in much repute, and all the species were considered useful in aiding parturition, from which they have acquired the name of Birth-wort, and from their imaginary power of being complete antidotes to the poison of snakes, is to be attributed their vernacular term snake-root. All the species are of curious structure; many of them are hardy and climbing; thirty-one species are enumerated by Loudon.

The root of the *Aristolochia serpentaria* is very highly valued in America, as a remedy for the bites of poisonous serpents. In Europe it is used as an aromatic tonic, and it does not possess virtues superior to many of its class. It is used as a gargle in putrid sore throat, and it is given in the lower stages of fever to support the strength. Its virtues depend in a great measure on the essential oil which it contains.

ANGULAR-LEAVED CONTRAYERVA

Dorstenia contrayerva

Class and Order, Tetrandria Monogynia. Nat. Ord. Urticeæ.
Gen. Char. *Receptacle* fleshy, round or angular, in which the solitary seeds are situated.

Root perennial, knotty, fibrous; leaves on long foot-stalks, palmate, with five, seven, or more lobes, all radical; flower-stems erect, round, three or four inches high, terminated by the fleshy quadrangular receptacle, in which the flowers are imbedded; these are in some antheriferous, and in others pistiliferous; it is a native of South America and the West Indian islands; two other species, *D. houstonia* and *D. drekena*, are said to possess similar virtues, and the root of the three species are indiscriminately gathered and exported as Contrayerva.

Contrayerva is an aromatic tonic. It is seldom prescribed in Europe, but is a favourite remedy in the Brazils; it is employed in fevers, especially in those which are commonly called nervous; in dysentery, in general debility, and as a remedy for the bites of poisonous reptiles. Many authors have extolled this root as a most valuable medicine, but experience has not confirmed their favourable report.

WINTER'S BARK

Drymis winteri

Class and Order, Polyandria Tetragynia. Nat. Ord. Wintereæ.
Gen. Char. *Calix* two or three-cleft; *Petals* six to twelve; *Stamens* club-shaped; *Anthers* two-lobed; *Style* wanting; *Berries* clustered; *Seeds* disposed in two rows.

The tree producing Winter's bark is one of the largest growing on the inhospitable shores of Terra del Fuego, attaining to the height of fifty feet. It is an evergreen; the leaves placed alternately; flowers small, white, odorous; berries ovate, spotted. It has an agreeable aromatic taste, between that of Cinnamon and *Canella alba*, and was considered by Linnæus as the bark of the last named plant, but was described by Forster, who accompanied Captain Cook, under the name of Drymis, which is retained by Decandolle, who has described four other species of the genus.

At Fig. 3 I have drawn a specimen I found in the late Dr Rutherford's collection of barks, bearing the name *Wintera granatensis*. Its taste is more pungent than the true Winter's bark, but I have no particulars from whence it was procured. "The bark of *D. granatensis*, called *Casca d'Anta* in Brazil, is much used against colic; it is tonic, aromatic, and stimulant, and resembles, in nearly all respects, the *D. winteri* or Winter's bark."—*Plantes Usuelles*, 26–28. Fig. 1 was drawn from a fine specimen in the same collection, marked "*Wintera aromatica*, true, from the Straits of Magellan." Fig. 2, which represents the bark after the removal of the epidermis, was from the Materia Medica Museum.

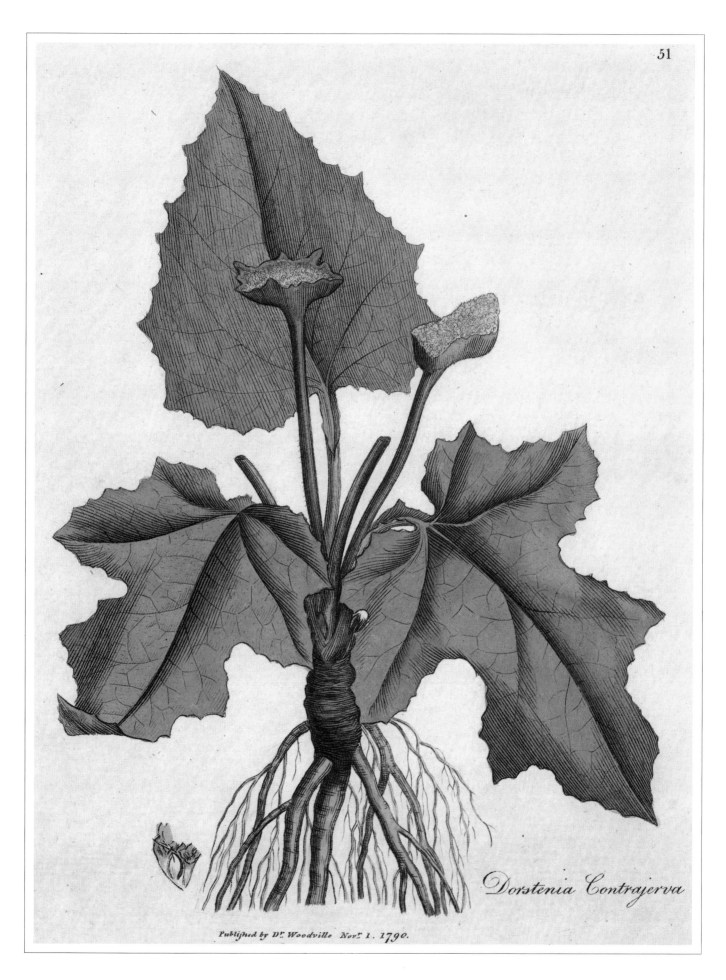

Dorstenia Contrajerva

Published by D.ʳ Woodville Nov.ʳ 1. 1790.

ANGULAR-LEAVED CONTRAYERVA

Winter's bark is a valuable aromatic stimulant and tonic; but it does not possess any properties which render it superior to others of its class. It forms an admirable addition to the simple bitters, such as gentian, quassia, or calumba; continental physicians frequently prescribe it. Canella is often substituted for Winter's bark, and the fraud is a very harmless one, as the virtues of each are the same.

CARIBEÆAN EXOSTEMMA

Exostemma caribea

Class and Order, Pentandria Monogynia. Nat. Ord. Rubiaceæ.
Gen. Char. *Calix* five-toothed; *Corolla* monopetalous, funnel-shaped; *Limb* five-parted, hairy; *Stamens* protruding; *Capsule* oblong, rounded, two-celled; *Seeds* numerous, with a membranous edge.

This genus was separated from Cinchona by Decandolle, and formed into a distinct genus,—the distinguishing features of which are the limb of the corolla being thickly clothed with pubescence, and the stamens protruding, which in all the true cinchonas are included in the tube of the flower. Besides these botanical discrepancies, this species differs in its medicinal properties, and would rather class with emetics than tonics. In external appearance, it differs materially from the cinchona bark; it is of a dark, blackish purple colour, having an exceedingly rough epidermis; and is totally devoid of the aromatic flavour that accompanies the officinal cinchonas. It was introduced from the West Indies in 1780, but has never been held in estimation in this country; it is sometimes found broken into small pieces, intermixed with the true drug, and is said to enter largely into the mixture of the various kinds when sent to the drug-mill. Fig. 4 was drawn from the Materia Medica Museum; Fig. 5 and 6 from those of Dr Rutherford.

The bark of the Exostemma is tonic and astringent, but it is seldom used. It occurs as a home adulteration of Peruvian bark, from which it is distinguished by chemical analysis, as well as by its therapeutic qualities. It contains no proximate principle; at least none has as yet been discovered.

COMMON MONKSHOOD, OR WOLFSBANE

Aconitum napellus

Class and Order, Polyandria Pentagynia. Nat. Ord. Ranunculaceæ.
Gen. Char. *Calix* five petal-like, irregular parts, the upper one concave and helmet-shaped, containing two pedunculated nectaries.

Root perennial, fusiform; stem from two to four feet high, leafy; leaves deeply cut, of a full shining green; flowers in spikes of a pale blue colour, sometimes quite smooth, at others thickly covered with hairs, which are particularly long on the veins and edges of the petals.

The plant varies considerably as to pubescence and colour; in some seasons being of a deep blue, and in succeeding years becoming of a pale violet or almost white. It is often found wild growing on river banks and on the banks of the same water course, I have found also the *Iris siberica, germanica*, and *gramineus*, and a large patch of *Hemerocallis flava*, the yellow day-lily, which in all probability have been thrown from some garden; in these wet conditions the flowers appear of a paler hue, and more pubescent than when growing in drier places.

The monkshood is among the most poisonous of plants, every part being deletrious; even the effluvia from the flowers are said to be narcotic. Numerous instances are on record of the fatal effects that have followed from eating the plant; one instance that fell under my notice, was that of a labouring gardener, who had been digging up the roots of Jerusalem artichokes for supper, and had inadvertently taken those of the present plant with them, to which they bear a considerable resemblance when not in a growing state. The roots were boiled and eaten by the gardener, to whom they proved fatal, and by another person who was an inmate of the same house; about a quarter of an hour after the roots were swallowed both the men complained of a burning sensation in the throat, which was not allayed by drinking plentifully of water; this symptom was followed by violent pains in the stomach and bowels, convulsive contractions of the face and limbs; these were speedily followed by insensibility; medical aid was called in about half an hour after the effects above-mentioned appeared, and emetics freely given; in the fatal

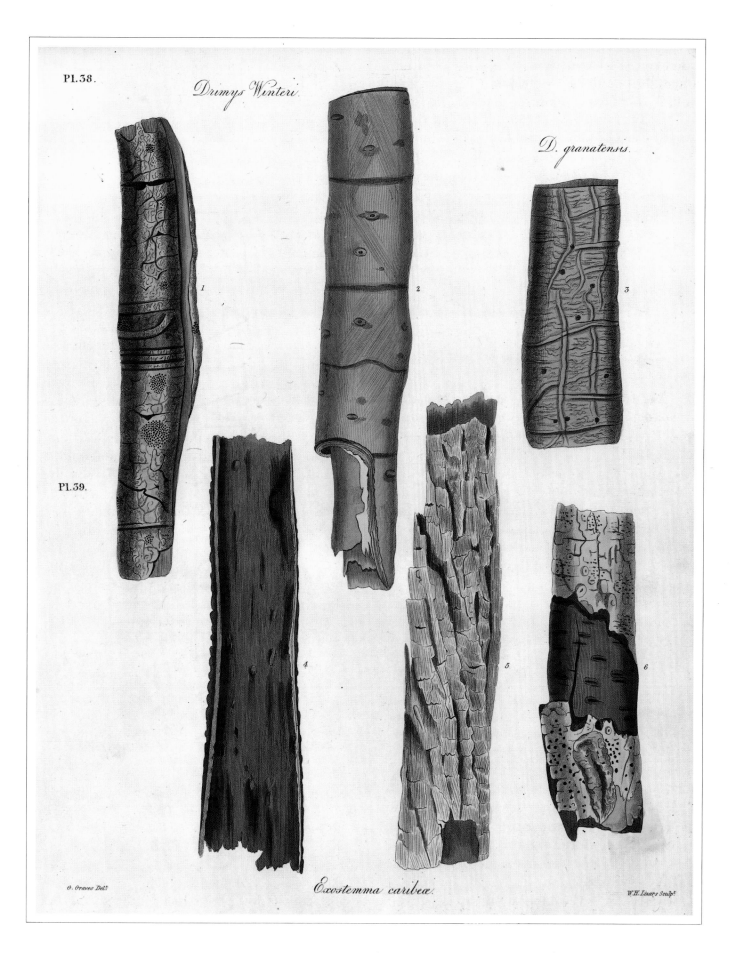

Pl. 38.

Drimys Winteri.

D. granatensis.

1

2

3

Pl. 39.

4

5

6

G. Graves Delt.

Exostemma caribea.

W.H. Lizars Sculpt.

WINTER'S BARK

case, without any effect; in the other, soap and water caused violent retching and a free evacuation of the bowels, after which the man appeared sinking, but upon administering warm brandy and water, from time to time, gradually recovered, but it was several weeks before he was able to return to his accustomed labour. About an hour after the food had been eaten, the man who died became strongly convulsed, with continued distortions of the limbs and countenance, the teeth and hands were clenched, the eyes partly closed, and the face of a livid purple, with white blotches; all attemps at relieving the stomach failed, and he died within three hours, without having been relieved by any evacuation. A *post mortem* examination was not permitted by the relatives of the deceased, but from the pain evidently endured much inflammation must have existed.

All the species of Aconite appear to possess similar properties; it is doubtful whether the present species, the *neomontanum* or the *paniculatum* is the true officinal, but from the identity of their properties, there can be little doubt but they may be indiscriminately applied to the same purposes. Of the extra-European kinds, the most virulent is probably the *A. ferox* figured by Dr Wallich, who gives the following interesting information: "There are three other species of *Aconitum* or monkshood, all of them tuberous-rooted, which inhabit the southern side of the Himalaya, and are considered as strong poisons by the natives." There is one in particular which contains a most virulent poison: "This dreadful root, of which large quantities are annually imported, is equally fatal when taken into the stomach, or applied to wounds, and is in universal use for poisoning arrows; and, there is too much reason to suspect, for the worst of purposes. Its importation would indeed seem to require the attention of the magistrates. The Gorkhalese pretent that it is one of their principal securities against invasion from the low countries; and that they would so infect all the waters, on the route by which an enemy was advancing, as to occasion his certain destruction. In case of such an attempt, the invaders ought no doubt to be on their guard; but the country abounds so in springs that might be soon cleared, as to render such a means of defence totally ineffectual, were the enemy aware of the circumstance. This poisonous species is called Bish or Bikh and Hadaya Bish or Bikh; nor am I certain whether the Metha ought to be referred to it, or to the foregoing kind."

Several species of aconite have been officinal at different times. The whole genus is poisonous, and several cases of poisoning are recorded. When a small quantity of the leaves is chewed, numbness of the lips and tongue followed by a sensation of pricking, is produced. In cases of poisoning with aconite, the symptoms are sometimes those of pure narcotic poisoning, at others they resemble those of acrid poisoning; sometimes maniacal delirium is present; in other cases the sensorium is not affected. Baron Stoerk introduced this plant as a remedy in chronic rheumatism, and other painful diseases of the neuralgic type; he likewise prescribed it in cancer, scrofula, and syphilis. The only pharmaceutic preparation of the aconite, in addition to the powered leaves, which is used in Britain, is the extract,—a very uncertain preparation; on the continent, the tincture and wine of the seeds are officinal. The powder of the leaves is perhaps the best form in which we can exhibit it, and the dose ought to be slowly increased, and the effects carefully watched, as it is a remedy which requires to be given in all cases with the greatest caution. Brandes and Peschier have published an account of the discovery of a vegetable alkaloid in Aconite. I have found a poisonous empyreumatic oil, which, I believe owes its properties to a volatile poisonous principle, similar to that of tobacco, hyoscyamus, &c.

PALMA CHRISTI OR CASTOR-OIL PLANT.

Ricinus communis

Class and Order, MONŒCIA MONADELPHIA. NAT. ORD. EUPHORBIACEÆ.
Gen. Char. Male; *Calix* five-parted; *Corolla* wanting; *Stamens* numerous.
Female; *Calix* three-parted; *Corolla* wanting; *Styles* three, bifid; *Capsule* three-celled; *Seed* one.

———

THIS species is an annual, which, under favourable circumstances, sometimes attains the height of twelve to sixteen feet, but which rarely exceeds that of three or four. When well-grown it is one of the most magnificent annual border plants. I raised one from seed sown on a heap of earth that had been dug out from six to seven

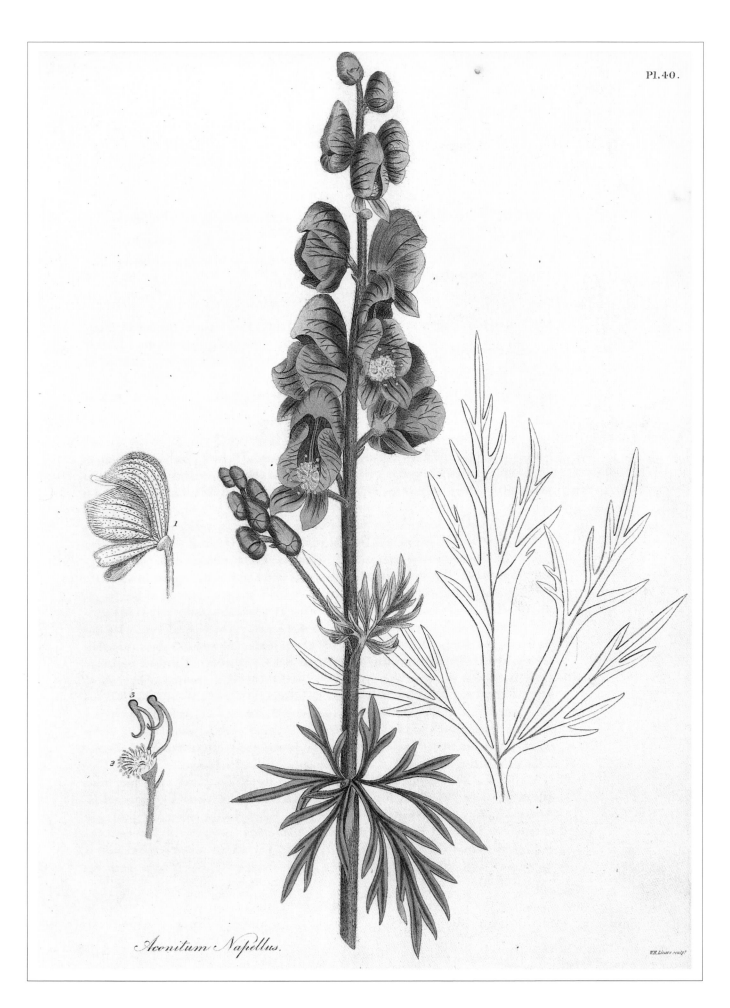

Aconitum Napellus.

Pl.40.

Aconitum Napellus.

COMMON MONKSHOOD OR WOLFSBANE; FIG.1, A FLOWER; FIG.2, NECTARIES AND
STAMENS AFTER REMOVING THE PERIANTH.

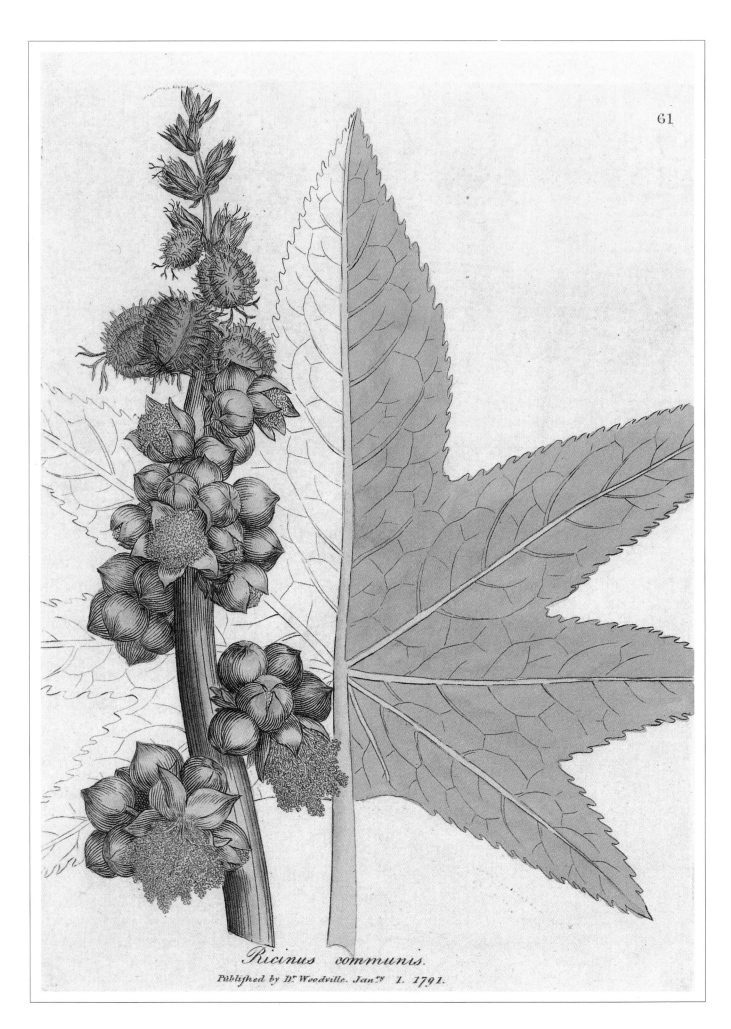

Ricinus communis.

Published by D.ᵣ Woodville. Jan.ʳʸ 1. 1791.

PALMA CHRISTI OR CASTOR-OIL PLANT

feet beneath the surface: the seed was deposited in the soil the second week in May; at the end of June it had acquired the height of three, and in August that of fifteen feet. The stem was four inches in diameter at the surface of the ground; and one of its largest leaves measured more than thirty inches from the insertion of the stalk to the point of the middle lobe. It flowered in September, and ripened its seeds the following month. I gathered more than two pints of ripe seeds, and there were upwards of twenty bunches of unripe ones at the time. The seeds were acrid and very oily. On the setting in of the frost, which was about the beginning of November, the lower leaves began to fall, but the flowers continued to open successively till the end of the year. The stem was covered with a thick coat of bloom, so much so as to appear as if covered with powdered blue.

In its native countries, the *Palma Christi* is a perennial plant, somewhat frutescent, and grows so tall as to require a ladder to collect its deeds; is a native of both the Indies, South America, China, various parts of the south of Spain, and opposite coasts of Africa, and some of the islands in the Mediterranean sea.

It was well known to the ancients and used by them as a cathartic,—the seeds being swallowed entire for that purpose; these are singularly marked, and bear a strong resemblance to an insect, from which circumstance it derives its name of *Ricinus*, a tick.

Nearly the whole of the plants belonging to the Euphorbiaceæ possess active properties.— some as cathartics, others as emetics, and a considerable number are virulent poisons. Among them is the famous manchineel-tree, *Hippomane mancinella*, which is said to be so poisonous that persons have died from merely sleeping beneath its shade, which, as Professor Lindley remarks, "is not so improbable as it may appear, when the volatile nature of the poisonous principle of these plants is considered."

Castor-oil, so well known as a purgative, is procured by expression, and by decoction. According to Dr Ainslie, that procured by decoction is the clearest and best-looking, and the most common. According to Dr Thomson, that obtained by pressure is much to be preferred. The seeds, from which the oil is obtained, are acrid, and purge with great violence. Their activity seems to depend on an acrid acid, which is volatile, and which is apt to get mixed with the oil when heat is employed in its preparation. In all cases in which a mild and strong purgative is desired, castor-oil ought to be employed; it evacuates the bowels freely, and removes any acrid matter with which they may have been loaded. In diarrhœa, and in the first stages of cholera, castor-oil, combined with opium, is very useful; in poisoning with the acrids, it is the only purgative which can be employed with safety. It can be given to the youngest infants, and to the most delicate females. The only objection to its use, is the sickness to which it gives rise, and this may generally be obviated by combining it with an aromatic, or by forming it into an emulsion. When combined with turpentine, it directs the action of that remedy to the intestines, and improves its action; the combination is an excellent vermifuge.

VIRGINIAN TOBACCO

Nicotiana tabacum

Class and Order, Pentandria Monogynia. Nat. Ord. Solaneæ.
Gen. Char. *Corolla* funnel-shaped; *Stigma* capitate; *Capsule* two-celled.

Tobacco was introduced into Britain from America in the year 1570, and from being an article of extreme luxury, has, by constant use, now almost become one of necessity. To persons who have accustomed themselves to its use, either in the form of snuff, smoke, or as a masticatory, its deprivation is attended with serious inconvenience. The present plant is an annual of ready growth and showy appearance, and is an ornament to the flower border. For domestic purposes, cultivators are allowed to grow it to the extent of half a rood; but, as an encouragement to our colonies, it is not permitted to be grown in larger quantities.

Root annual; stems erect, round, slightly grooved, branching at the top; leaves numerous, alternate, pointed, entire,—the lower ones often attaining two feet in length, and from four to six inches in breadth; flowers green at the base of the tube, gradually enlarging, and expanding into five deep rose-coloured segments. The whole plant is covered with a clammy down, which is exceedingly fetid, and every part is strongly narcotic. The same properties pervade the whole of this genus, of which twenty-four species and nine varieties are mentioned in Loudon's Hortus Britannicus.

Notwithstanding the attempts of almost every government both in Europe and Asia, and the severe punishments with which they menaced all those who used tobacco either in the form of snuff or smoke, we find it now habitually used by a very large proportion of the inhabitants of Europe, Asia, and America. It was brought to Britain by Sir Walter Raleigh in the reign of Elizabeth, and in the following reign its use had become so prevalent, that James the VI. published against it under the title of "The Counterblaste to Tobacco;" and the same monarch proposed as a banquet for the devil, "a loin of pork, a poll of ling, and a pipe of tobacco for digestion." There can be no doubt that the habit of taking any stimulus constantly is injurious, and we know well that tobacco is a stimulus in whatever way it is taken, though in some forms its stimulant properties soon yield to its sedative. Dr Thomson considers snuffing as the least injurious mode of using tobacco; and he considers the statements with regard to its baneful effects as being greatly exaggerated. In the snuff-manufactories of France, where 4000 persons are employed, it has been ascertained that they live as long, and are as healthy, as manufacturers in general. Smoking produces very different effects on different constitutions,— some get readily habituated to it, while others suffer from nausea, vertigo, vomiting, and general depression. Smoking to excess destroys the tone of the stomach, and causes general emaciation. Tobacco is used medicinally as an errhine, in the form of snuff; as a sedative and expectorant, in the form of smoke; and as an antispasmodic, stimulant, and sedative, in the form of infusion. It is not so well adapted for an errhine as many other substances, on account of its narcotic properties. As a sedative, it is given both by the mouth, and as an enema in the form of smoke; but this form is objectionable, as it is not very manageable, and as the effects come on with great rapidity. As an expectorant, it is useful in those habits where its depressing and nauseating effects are not readily produced, and where inflammatory symptoms are absent. In the form of infusion, it acts, when taken internally in very small doses, as a diuretic. When given as a glyster, it acts as a stimulant in doses of seven or eight grains; in larger doses it acts as a sedative or antispasmodic, and is frequently used in strangulated hernia, in obstinate constipation, and in ileus.

In cholera, the infusion was proposed as a stimulating, antispasmodic enema, and very sanguine anticipations were formed of its success. I tried it in several cases, but did not find that any permanently favourable result followed.

COMMON HENBANE

Hyoscyamus niger

Class and Order, Pentandria Monogynia. Nat. Ord. Solaneæ.
Gen. Char. *Calix* tubular, five-clefted; *Corolla* funnel-shaped, oblique; *Capsule* two-celled, opening with a lid.

The Henbane is usually of biennial duration, but very frequently only survives the first year; it grows wild in most areas, and like many other plants that are commonly cultivated, has probably been originally cast out from gardens. It grows on sandy and chalky soils, usually in the vicinity of towns or villages, as also on the sea shore; the largest I remember to have met with in a wild state grew by the road side to a height of five or six feet, and was branched from the bottom; all the waste ground in that neighbourhood produced Henbane in abundance.

Root fusiform, thick, succulent, wrinkled, fibrous; stems from one to three or four feet high, much branched, round; leaves deeply sinuate; calix veined, the bottom part swollen and enclosing the capsule, from which when ripe the lid or upper part falls off. The whole plant is covered with viscid fetid hairs, which are more dense and longer on the globular part of the calix. The whole plant gives out a heavy peculiar odour, which is highly narcotic. The other species are said to possess the same medical properties as the present one; twelve are mentioned in *Loudon's Encyclopedia*.

Hyoscyamus is perhaps, after opium, the most valuable narcotic in our Materia Medica; it agrees with most constitutions, and does not in general cause that depression and nausea which follow the sleep induced by opium; it also acts as a gentle laxative. I have found it when combined with a diaphoretic, one of the best remedies in those slight febrile attacks which accompany

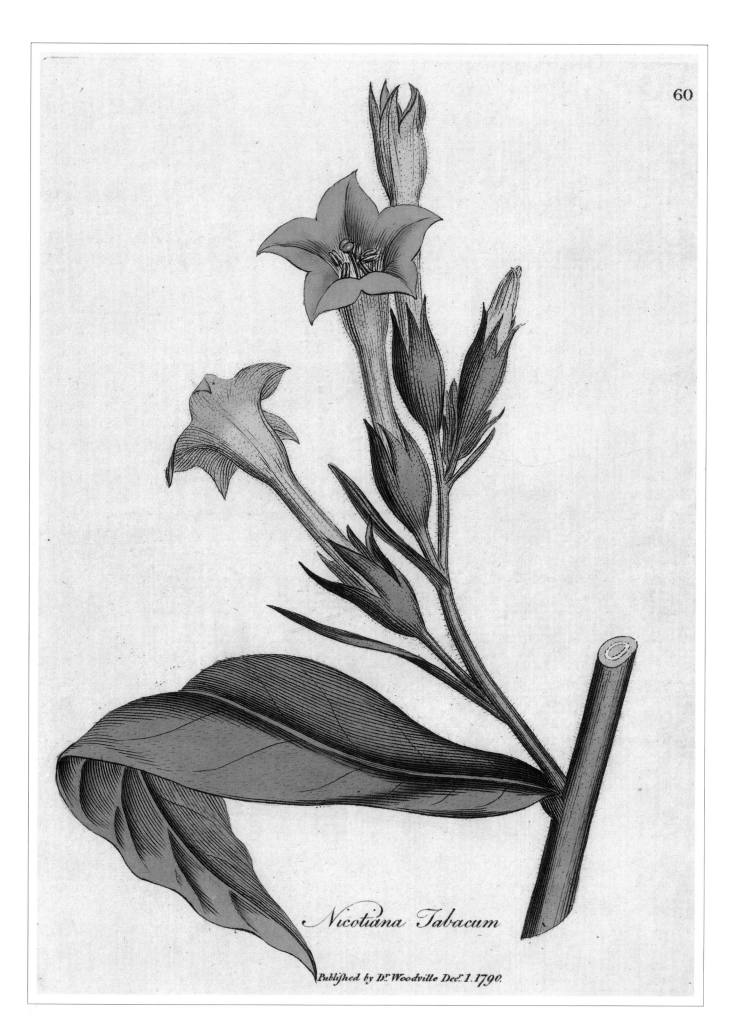

Nicotiana Tabacum

Published by Dr Woodville Decr 1. 1790.

VIRGINIAN TOBACCO

common colds in some habits. Combined with aloes and soap, it is well known as "Hamilton's Female Pill," one of the best and mildest purgatives for habitual use. Like Belladonna, it possesses the property of causing dilation of the pupil, and of giving relief in ophthalmia.

PIMENTO OR ALLSPICE

Pimenta vulgaris

Class and Order, Icosandria Monogynia. Nat. Ord. Myrtaceæ.
Gen. Char. *Calix* of five segments; *Petals* five; *Ovary* two-celled; *Ovules* solitary, appense; *Style* straight; *Stigma* somewhat capitate.

This species was separated from the genus *Myrtus* by Professor Lindley, from the difference in the structure of its fruit; is a native of the West Indies, where it is an evergreen tree, growing to the height of thirty feet; it produces its flowers at the extremities of the branches in large loose bunches; they are pale greenish-yellow, and are followed by purple berries, each containing two seeds; as soon as they are nearly ripe they are gathered, and either dried in the sun or by artificial means; when perfectly dry they are packed for exportation.

The Pimento berries or Allspice belong to the same class of remedies with the clove, cinnamon, and nutmeg. They derive their name of Allspice from combining the flavour of these aromatics, and they may be used as a substitute for any or all of them in practice. They are not, however, much used in medicine, but are frequently taken as condiments.

CLOVE-TREE

Caryophyllus aromaticus

Class and Order, Icosandria Monogynia. Nat. Ord. Myrtaceæ.
Gen. Char. *Calix* funnel-shaped, four-parted; *Petals* four; *Germen* two-celled, oblong, fruit dry, one or two-celled.

The Clove-tree is a native of the Moluccas, but is extensively cultivated in the West Indies, China, the East Indies, as well as the adjacent islands. The tree grows to the height of forty or more feet, and is branched almost from the bottom; the whole tree is aromatic, but the buds or unexpanded flowers are the officinal part, and are the well-known spice. Few clove plants are in Britain, nor does it thrive so well as many other tropical trees. The leaves are long, pointed, and placed on a foot-stalk, which is said to be the most aromatic part of the plant; the flowers grow in clusters at the extremity of the branches, are of a yellowish green colour, tinged with red, which is stronger on the tubular part of the calix, and often is of a purple tinge. When fresh, the spice has a somewhat unctuous feel, and when fine, the petals should be persistent on the crown of the calix; they are often adulterated by the admixture of others, from which the oil has been extracted, which may be detected by the lightness of their weight and colour; and if an incision be made in them, they appear quite dry, whilst in the sound and perfect spice the oil appears upon the puncture of a pin. This is the only species.

Of the aromatic excitants, cloves are perhaps the most powerful and certain; they require, however, to be given with caution, as they are apt to cause vertigo, headache, and other disagreeable symptoms, when given in an overdose. The essential oil of cloves is extremely active; its taste is warm, aromatic and acrid; when taken undiluted, it causes a burning sensation in the mouth and fauces, and small vesications are frequently formed. In cholera, I found that the oils of cloves, cinnamon, and nutmeg, as well as those of peppermint and cajeput, were retained on the stomach when nothing else would remain, and I observed that the stimulation of the system by them was more permanent and more beneficial, than that produced by alcohol or ether. Bonastre has examined oil of cloves, and has discovered a crystalline substance, which he calls *Caryophylline*, but which appears to be a variety of *Stearoptêne*. Nitric acid strikes a deep red colour with oil of cloves, and we are warned not to confound it with that of strychnia or morphia in medico-legal investigation. Oil of cloves is very useful in alleviating toothache.

CINNAMON

Laurus cinnamomum

Class and Order, Enneadria Monogynia. Nat. Ord. Laurineæ.
Gen. Char. *Calix* four to six-parted; *Nectariferous glands* three, with two bristles surrounding the *ovary*; *Anthers* opening transversely; *Valves* hinged to the upper side.

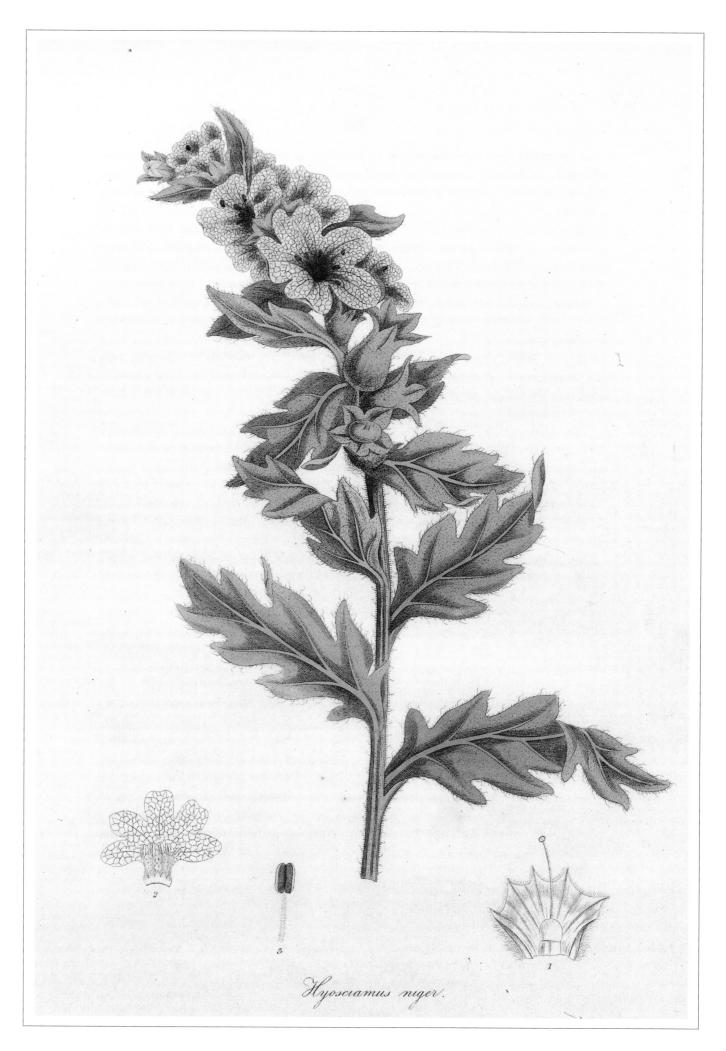

Hyosciamus niger.

COMMON HENBANE

THIS valuable spice-tree is a native of Ceylon, Malabar, Cochin-China, and Sumatra, and is cultivated in the Mauritius, and some of the West India islands. The *Laurus cinnamomum*, or true cinnamon, is a tree about twenty or thirty feet high, with numerous suckers from the root. The leaves are large, pointed, opposite, growing in pairs, with very prominent nerves, which disappear as they approach the point; the young leaves and stems are at first deep-red, but, as they acquire their full growth, become of a full green. The flowers are both axillary and terminal, of a sullied white colour, and are succeeded by deep purple berries, which are a favourite food with crows and wood-pigeons. It very closely resembles the *L. cassia*, which has longer and narrower leaves, with a less agreeable taste, the bark of which is frequently substituted for that of the true cinnamon, than which it is much heavier, and breaks short, whereas the cinnamon has an irregular and splintering fracture.

Cinnamon is the bark of the young branches, which are cut off and carefully peeled. After the bark is freed from its epidermis, and any parts of the wood that might have been removed in decorticating the stems, the smaller pieces are placed within the larger quills. It soon dries, and is made up in bundles, and, previous to exportation, is examined by government officers to ascertain its quality. It usually comes to the British market in small bundles of one or two pounds weight. Cinnamon of the best quality is of a fine reddish-yellow colour, of a very thin texture, of a sweetish full flavour, and is distinguished from cassia by being thinner, lighter, of a brighter colour, and having a flavour pungent, but not fiery, as in that species. The article known in the druggist's shops under the name of cassia buds, are the fleshy receptacles of the seed of this plant.

Cinnamon is one of the most agreeable excitants which we possess; it is seldom used alone, but forms a grateful addition to bitter infusions or powders. The volatile oil is extremely pungent, warm, and aromatic, and it has a peculiar sweetness; the oil of cassia which is obtained from the coarser bark of the cinnamon tree, resembles oil of cinnamon in flavour, but it is not so agreeable. The oil of cinnamon is liable to adulteration from its great price, and the oil of cassia is generally used for this purpose, as it is much cheaper, and as it cannot be easily detected. The leaves of the *Laurus cinnamomum* contain an oil closely resembling that of cloves.

TRUE NUTMEG-TREE

Myristica moschata

Class and Order, DIŒCIA MONADELPHIA. NAT. ORD. MYRISTICEÆ.

Gen. Char. Male flower: *Calix* wanting; *Corolla* campanulate, trifid; *Filaments* united into a columnar tube; *Anthers* six or ten, cohering at the base.
Female flower: *Calix* wanting; *Corolla* campanulate, trifid; *Stigmas* two; *Berry* with an arilled one-seeded nut; *Seed* large, veiny, variegated on the inside.

THE nutmeg is a native of the Moluccas or Spice islands, and has been introduced into the isles of France, Bourbon, and Sumatra, also to our West Indian colonies; to St Vincents, it was brought from Cayenne, and the trees which were originally imported have attained a considerable size, but the nutmeg does not appear to succeed so well in the West as in the East Indies. Dr Hooker has given beautiful representations of both sexes of this valuable tree, first in his splendid Exotic Flora, and afterwards in the Botanical Magazine, with a highly interesting history of the plant, to which I must refer such of my readers as wish to become more particularly acquainted with the details of its political as well as botanical history.

In the Moluccas, it grows to the height of twenty or thirty feet, and is clothed with numerous oblong, pointed, smooth leaves, of a full shining green, with small bunches of pale yellow flowers growing from the axils of the leaves; it blossoms throughout the year, bearing ripe fruit and flowers at the same time; the fruit when at maturity is as large as a moderate sized pear, and of a similar form, of a reddish-yellow colour on the outside, within nearly white; this when ripe splits in the centre, and exposes the *arillus* or mace with which the nut is enveloped, which is of a brilliant scarlet colour, and very glossy; beneath this is a thin hard shell containing the nutmeg, which when ripe is perfectly smooth, but on drying becomes shrivelled. The spice is gathered at three periods of the year; "in July and August, when the nutmegs are most abundant, but the mace is thinner than in the smaller fruits which are gathered during November, the second time of collecting. The third harvest takes place in the month of March or beginning of April, when the nuts as well as the mace are in the greatest perfection, their number being then not so great, and the season dry. The outer pulpy coat is removed, and afterwards the mace with a knife. The nuts are placed over a slow fire, when the shell becomes brittle, and the seeds or nutmegs drop out; these are then soaked in sea water and impregnated with lime, a process which answers the double purpose of securing the seeds from the attack of insects, and of destroying their vegetating property. It further prevents the volatilization of the aroma. The mace is simply dried in the sun, and then sprinkled with salt water, after which it is fit for exportation."

The best nuts are heavy, firm, of a gray colour externally, within beautifully marbled with red and brown; the mace is at first of a brilliant scarlet, but when dried of a deep saffron colour. The oil, usually denominated oil of mace, is expressed from the small or imperfect nutmegs; it is imported in small earthen jars, is soft, of a yellow colour, having the fragrance of the nutmeg. There are several inferior sorts, and all are liable to adulteration; the best is free from impurities, of a bright colour, and very fragrant.

A few specimens of the tree are now in Britain; but as they require the constant temperature of the stove to bring them to perfection, we can scarcely hope to see them flower in Britain.

The nutmeg is a warm, aromatic, stimulant tonic, and is used for the same purposes as cinnamon. It contains an essential and a fixed oil, which are obtained by distillation and expression.

SWEET-BAY

Laurus nobilis

Class and Order, Natural Order and Generic Character, see *L. Cinnamomum.*

THE Sweet-Bay is a handsome evergreen shrub, and highly ornamental, and, though a native of Italy and Greece, bears the cold of climates more northern without injury. In its native soil it rises to the height of twenty or thirty feet, but in Britain only forms a low bushy shrub, with numerous suckers surrounding the stem; its leaves are a deep shining green, pale beneath,

the edges undulated; the plants are unisexual, and have their racemes of white flowers on short pedicels; these are only produced in sheltered situations. Its leaves are occasionally used in culinary preparations.

The berries of the laurel yield on expression a greenish oil, which is occasionally used as an external application. Its virtues depend on the presence of volatile oil, which is aromatic, warm, and stimulant.

SASSAFRAS-TREE

Laurus sassafras

Class and Order, Natural Order, and Generic Character, see *L. Cinnamomum.*

THIS species is common to North America, and bears our climate uninjured; it forms a handsome tree of large dimensions. The leaves that first appear are entire and pointed; these are succeeded by others having only one lobe, but those that follow are constantly with three lobes; the flowers are short pendant stalks, and are placed in interrupted whorls round the stems.

Sassafras is a stimulant diaphoretic, and is much used in secondary syphilis. The infusion is the best form of exhibition; for its virtues depend in a great measure on the presence of volatile oil, the decoction becomes much less active. Both the root and wood are used in medicine; the root contains about three per cent. of volatile oil, and is much more active than the wood. The volatile oil is colourless when recent, but it acquires a yellowish red by keeping; it is warm and pungent to the taste; and its odour is rather agreeable.

CAMPHOR-TREE

Laurus camphora

Class and Order, Nat. Ord. and Generic Character, see *L. Cinnamomum.*

THOUGH the larger part of the camphor of commerce is obtained from this species, camphor is a constituent part of a very considerable number of plants of various families. Camphor laurel is a native of Japan, and forms a large tree with long lanceolate leaves and small white flowers. The camphor is obtained from the stem and roots by distillation; it is also found in small grains, concreted in the grain of the wood, and sometimes as a pulverulent exudation on the surface of the leaves. A principle resembling it is likewise found in thyme, marjoram, rosemary, and numerous other plants; it is also to be procured from cinnamon, and probably from other species of laurel.

The *Dryabalanops camphora* is a very lofty tree, acquiring the height of nearly a hundred feet. Camphor is found in a concrete state in the trunks of the trees, which is ascertained by boring; when it is discovered, the tree is felled, and large masses of camphor, from ten to twenty pounds weight, are found at intervals in the heart of the stems.

To procure camphor, the roots, wood, and branches of the *Laurus camphora* are cut into small pieces, and put into a still with a quantity of water. When the water has boiled for forty-eight hours, the operation is considered complete, and the camphor is found adhering to the straw with which the head of the still is lined. In this state it is mixed with impurities, to free it from which, the Dutch, who import it, sublime it in glass vessels, having previously mixed it with a small portion of quicklime, to retain any empyreumatic oil which may be formed. When pure, camphor is white, crystalline, transparent, and somewhat unctuous to the touch, brittle, but tough and elastic, so as to be pulverized with the greatest difficulty; of an aromatic pungent bitterish taste, leaving a sensation of cold in the mouth. It has a peculiar penetrating odour, it is lighter than water, very volatile and inflammable, buring with a bright flame, without leaving any residuum.

Camphor is a powerful stimulant, and when given in very large doses acts as a poison, causing syncope, convulsions, and delirium; opium acts as an antidote. Camphor acts as a narcotic where opium has failed of success. It is a useful remedy in debility, in hysteria, in spasmodic affections, and in dyspepsia arising from flatulence. It is also said to correct the bad effects which are caused by an overdose of opium, mezereon, or cantharides, and it certainly often removes the disagreeable effects which sometimes follow the application of a blister. In indolent tumours, and in rheumatic affections, a liniment containing camphor in solution is often of service.

CHAMOMILE

Anthemis nobilis

Class and Order, Syngenesia Superflua. Nat. Ord. Compositæ.
Gen. Char. *Involucre* hemispherical, imbricated with nearly equal scales, whose margins are membranaceous; *Receptacle* convex, chaffy; *Fruit* crowned with a membranaceous border or pappus.

Root perennial, frequently extending a foot or more on the surface of the ground, and throwing out fibres at distant parts, and these mostly from where the root is enlarged, and annularly jointed; stems six to ten inches long, trailing, and furrowed, which renders the stalks angular; lower leaves one or two inches long, with bi or tripinnate leaflets, which are nearly round; the leaves growing near the flower smaller,—often of only three divisions or pinnulæ; flowers terminal, white, but not unfrequently composed of florets without the exterior petals or rays.

Chamomile grows wild mostly in the vicinity of gardens or amongst rubbish. It is cultivated in great quantities for medicinal purposes; and a variety with double flowers has, to a considerable extent, supplanted the common sort; it has a more showy appearance, but is very inferior to the common chamomile,—its redundancy of petals by no means compensating for the loss of the fleshy receptacle, in which the particular virtue of the plant is said to reside. When intended for infusion, the flowers are to be preferred, but for all purposes of fomentation, the stems, leaves, and flowers, are of equal value. It is a hardy perennial of easy culture, which will grow in the most sterile soils, and is then more strongly impregnated with its peculiar aroma, than when in richer soils, where it attains to a larger size, and its flowers alter their appearance by producing almost exclusively petaloid florets, when the receptacle becomes much flattened, and loses a large portion of its fragrance.

Chamomile flowers are a very common and excellent remedy, and are often used with advantage in flatulent hysteric affections, and in cases where simple bitters and tonics are indicated. They contain bitter extractive and essential oil. Their tonic properties may be with plausibility attributed to the former, and their antispasmodic and carminative properties to the latter. The infusion, or chamomile tea, as it is

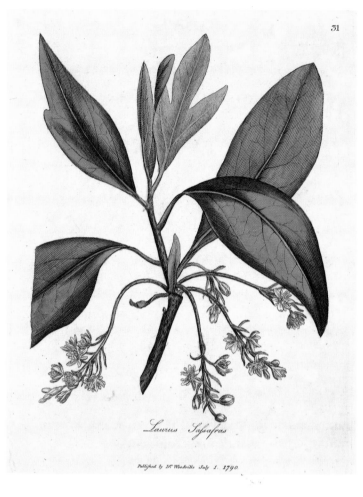

Laurus Sassafras

Published by Dr Woodville July 1. 1790.

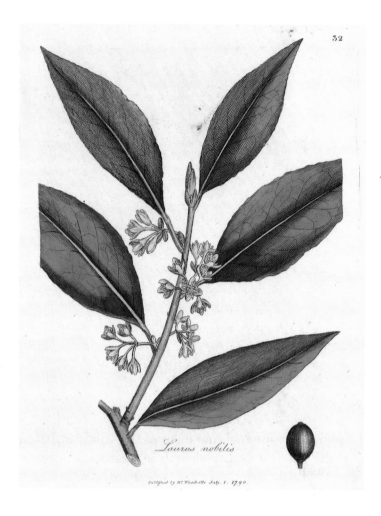

Laurus nobilis

Published by Dr Woodville July 1. 1790.

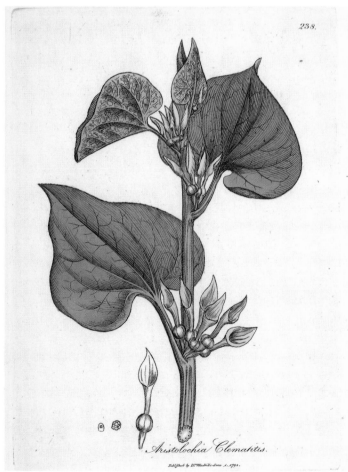

Aristolochia Clematitis.

Published by Dr Woodville June 1. 1791.

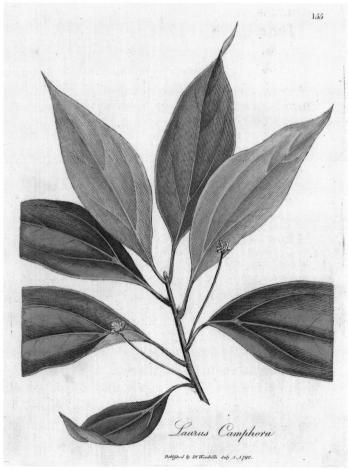

Laurus Camphora

Published by Dr Woodville July 1. 1792.

TOP LEFT: SASSAFRAS TREE, TOP RIGHT: SWEET BAY, BOTTOM LEFT: BIRTHWORT
OR VIRGINIAN SNAKE-ROOT, BOTTOM RIGHT: CAMPHOR TREE

called, is the best form of administering it. When given in very large doses, it causes vomiting, and it is a very common emetic among the country people.

PELLITORY OF SPAIN

Anthemis pyrethrum

Class and Order, Nat. Order, and Generic Character, see *A. nobilis.*

A hardy perennial of easy culture, and very ornamental in the flower border; it is a native of the south of Europe. The root is long, descending a foot or more, with lateral branches and fibres; leaves resembling those of chamomile but smaller; stems procumbent, about a foot long, with but few lateral ones; each is terminated with a large white flower, with the florets of the centre of a golden yellow; the back of each of the exterior flowers or rays with a purple stripe in the middle, and a yellow tinge at the base. The root, which is the drug of the shops, should be well dried, perfectly free from mouldiness, and of a pale brown colour; when held in the mouth a short time produces a burning sensation, which is not speedily removed.

The root of the *Anthemis pyrethrum* is used as a sialagogue; when chewed it creates a feeling of coldness, accompanied by a prickly sensation, and a very much increased flow of saliva. It is much used in toothach, which it occasionally relieves.

PEPPERMINT

Mentha piperita

Class and Order, Didynamia Gymnospermia. Nat. Ord. Labiatæ.
Gen. Char. *Calix* equal, five-toothed; mouth naked or rarely villous; *Corolla* nearly regular, of four segments; *Tube* very short; *Stamens distant*, protruding or included; *Filaments* naked; *Anthers* with two parallel cells.

Root perennial, creeping fibrous; stems erect, quadrangular, striated, branched at the top, rising from one or two feet in height; leaves sharply serrated, of a full green, opposite; flowers small, in dense clusters, growing in interrupted spikes.

The Peppermint grows naturally in watery places, but from its creeping roots, is likely to be an outcast from gardens. It is subject to considerable variety in the shape, and greater or less hairiness of its leaves; in dry exposed situations it becomes covered with a close soft pubescence, but in moist situations, is sparingly furnished with hairs, and those principally on the veins of the leaves. The Mints are numerous, but, from their varying in their appearance, the species are by no means easily determined; fifty-two species and six varieties are mentioned in Loudon.

Peppermint has a strong, rather agreeable odour, and a pungent aromatic taste. Its virtues reside in an essential oil of a pale yellowish-green colour, which is procured from it by distillation, in the proportion of about three and a-half ounces from twenty-five pounds of the fresh plant. In doses of from three to five drops, the oil is much used as a carminative. The distilled water and spirit are also given for the same purpose, and are very useful remedies in flatulence and anorexia, arising from loss of tone in the stomach. The oil forms a valuable addition to various purgative medicines, as it prevents griping. I found it beneficial in cholera, as it frequently remained on the stomach when no other stimulent was retained.

It is composed of a fluid and solid oil, considered by some chemists as a variety of camphor.

SPEARMINT

Mentha viridis

Class and Order, Nat. Ord. and Generic Character, see *M. pipertia.*

Root perennial, creeping, fibrous; stems erect, quadrangular; leaves longer than the preceding, and of brighter and paler colour; flowers purple, like those of the Peppermint, which the whole plant much resembles, excepting in the length of its foliage. Found wild in similar situations with the Peppermint, and is often the outcast of gardens; both this and the preceding species are cultivated to a considerable extent in various parts of England.

The *Mentha viridis* is seldom used medicinally. It yields a volatile oil resembling that of peppermint, but less agreeable. A distilled water is also prepared from it, but it is little used. For culinary purposes this mint is generally selected.

Pl.42.

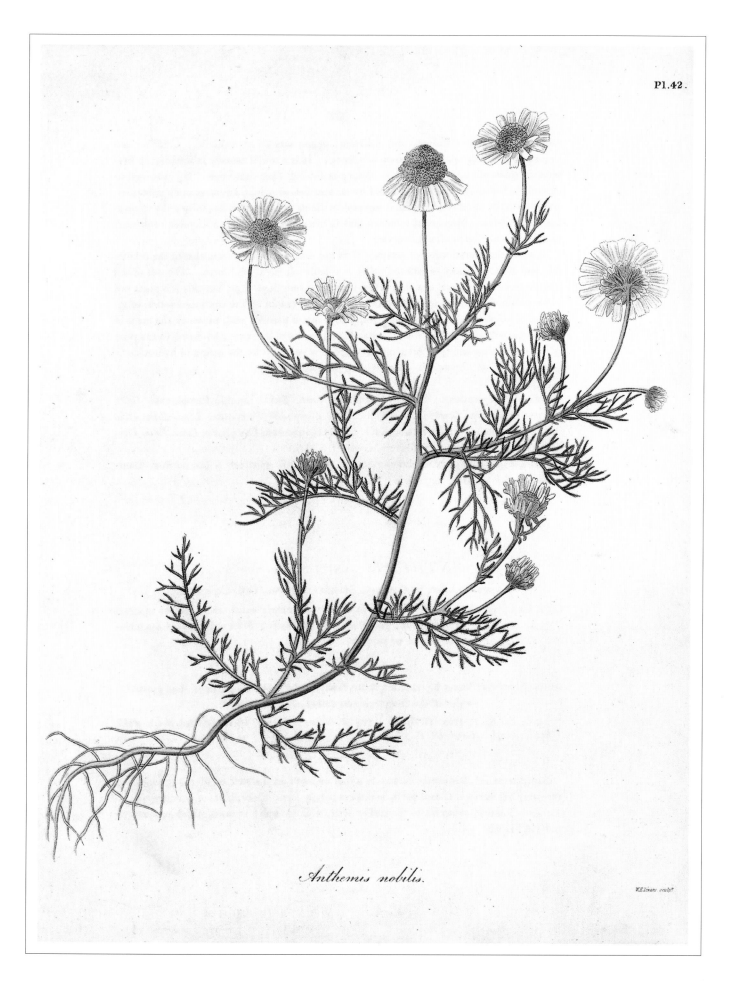

Anthemis nobilis.

W.E.Linars sculpt

CHAMOMILE

Pl. 45.

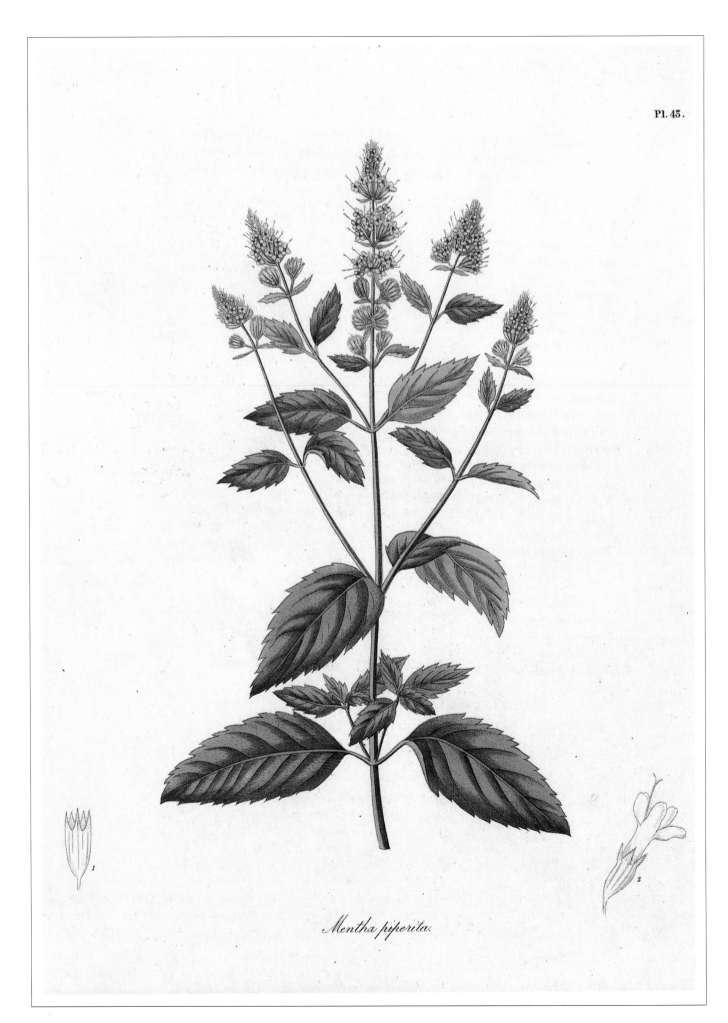

Mentha piperita.

PEPPERMINT; FIG.1, CALIX; FIG.2, FLOWER; BOTH MAGNIFIED

PENNY-ROYAL

Mentha pulegium

Class and Order, Nat. Ord. and Generic Character, see
M. piperita.

PENNY-ROYAL is the smallest of the family of mints; it is found usually in wet and marshy places. Root perennial, creeping, fibrous; stems prostrate, less quadrangular than the two preceding species; leaves obtuse, frequently recurved; flowers in whorls; the whole plant has a powerful odour.

Penny-royal is the most disagreeable of the mints. It contains essential oil, and may be used for all the purposes for which peppermint is usually employed.

COMMON HOP

Humulus lupulus

**Class and Order, DIŒCIA PENTANDRIA. NAT. ORD.
URTICEÆ.**
Gen. Char. Barren flower: *Perianth* of five leaves; *Anthers* with two pores at the extremity.
Fertile flower: *Scales* of the catkin large, persistent, concave, entire, single-flowered; *Perianth* wanting; *Styles* two; *Seed* one.

THE Hop is often met with in a wild state, growing luxuriantly in hedge-rows and coppices; but as it was more diffusedly cultivated before it became an exciseable article, it has probably been thrown out from gardens.

The Hop is a perennial, climbing, herbaceous plant; stems long, weak and scabrous; leaves on footstalks, three or five-lobed, deeply serrated, veiny and rough; flowers yellowish-green; fertile flowers resembling a pine-cone. This is the only known species.

The principal purpose to which hops are applied is in the manufacture of beer. Hops are among the most precarious crops the agriculturist has to do with, and it is calculated that every fifth year is an entire failure; the produce varies from two or three to twenty or twenty-five hundred-weight on the acre; the medium is accounted a remunerating crop. The plants require a deep rich well-manured soil; in some parts of Britain old woollen rags, blankets, and carpets, are used as manure, being ploughed in between the rows. In forming a hop plantation the ground requires to be well-cleared, and trenched deep either with the plough or spade, the young plants or sets are placed in a circle, six or seven in a patch, and the rows require to be at least six feet apart; there is but little produce till after the third year, when they come into full-bearing, and continue for twelve or fifteen years; the plantation requires constant attention, from the time the shoots emerge from the ground, until after the harvesting of the hops; as soon as the shoots appear they are secured to poles, which, for the first two years, are from six to eight feet high, but the next season they are supplied with poles fourteen or sixteen feet in length; and it is generally remarked, that, unless the hop-bine attains to the height of the poles by midsummer, a failure usually ensues; the plants are subject to injury from various insects, particularly from what is termed the fly, which commits its ravages so rapidly that a healthy plantation will in a short time after the appearance of this insect have all the indication of a premature winter; the leaves shrivel and become brown, and it but rarely happens that the plants recover.

The hop ripens about the end of August, or beginning of September, and being dried in a kiln similar to that used in malting, are packed in large sacks; the best kinds are put into smaller packages of a finer texture called pockets, which contain from one hundred to one hundred and thirty pounds each, but the bulk are packed in large coarse sacks, called bags, which will contain about three hundred-weight.

The young shoots of the hop are by some used as a substitute for asparagus; these are seldom taken but from the roots of the first or second year's planting.

The hop was at one time supposed to possess valuable narcotic properties, but the expectations of many on this head have been disappointed, and, as Dr A.T. Thomson says, "it can only be regarded as a pleasant bitter; the best mode of exhibiting it is in well-brewed beer; the Lupulin is a weak narcotic." *Lupulin*, as it has been called, is a compound of wax, tannin, bitter extractive, and volatile oil; and has therefore no pretensions to be called by the name *Lupulin*, which indicates that it is an active and distinct principle. Hops are supposed to render malt liquors less injurious, and they certainly retard the acetous fermentation, and consequently cause it to keep much longer than it would otherwise do. All malt liquor intended for exportation to warm climates is more highly hopped than that which is brewed for home consumption.

LOGWOOD

Hæmatoxylon campechianum

Class and Order, Decandria Monogynia. Nat. Ord. Leguminosæ.
Gen. Char. *Calix* five-parted; *Petals* five; *Capsule* lanceolate, one-celled, two-valved; *Valves* boat-shaped.

This tree, which produces the logwood of commerce, is the only known species. It is a native of South America, growing abundantly in the Bay of Campeachy, from whence it derives its specific name. It forms a low tree; stem crooked; leaves abruptly pinnate; flowers pale-yellow.

Logwood is one of our most valuable dyes, and is used for staining woods, which it dyes nearly black, with the addition of salts of iron.

Logwood is occasionally prescribed with advantage in chronic diarrhœa, but it is principally valuable as a dye.

RATTLESNAKE ROOT

Polygala senega

Class and Order, Diadelphia Octandria. Nat. Ord. Polygaleæ.
Gen. Char. *Calix* of five leaves, two of them wing-shaped and coloured; *Petals* combined by their claws with the filaments, the lower one keeled; *Capsule* compressed; *Seed* downy, crested at the hilum.

This species of Milkwort is common to most parts of North America, and, probably from the circumstance of its knotty root having some resemblance to the tail of the rattlesnake, may have induced the belief in its efficacy as a cure for the venom of that animal. It varies from white to rose-colour in its flowers; and having long been in cultivation, several varieties are mentioned, originating from the different modes of culture; it is a hardy perennial plant of ready growth. Decandolle enumerates more than one hundred and sixty species; one, *P. vulgaris*, and a second species, *P. amara*, has recently been found, but the specimens I have seen of this last kind I suspect to be only large grown plants of *vulgaris*; they both possess a peculiar taste, resembling the *senega*, but are more bitter; the *vulgaris* varies with white, red, purple and blue flowers.

Rattlesnake root is stimulant, diuretic, and expectorant, and is well adapted for the treatment of chronic catarrh, asthma, and hydrothorax. In Germany it is used as an internal remedy in ophthalmia. In America it is much extolled as an antidote to the poison of various reptiles, particularly of the rattlesnake. It is not extensively used in Britain, but some practitioners are very partial to it, and prescribe it as an adjunct in many chronic diseases. When inflammatory symptoms are acute, the stimulating properties of this plant render it unsafe.

SUMACH OR POISON-OAK

Rhus toxicodendron

Class and Order, Pentandria Trigynia. Nat. Ord. Anacardiaceæ.
Gen. Char. *Calix* five-parted; *Petals* five; *Berry* one-seeded.

This is an exceedingly poisonous plant, and its poison is not only communicated by touching or smelling it, but affects some persons who approach near the tree; to others it is innoxious. It is a native of North America, and was introduced into Europe in 1640.

Stem trailing, or, when supported, climbing in the manner of ivy; leaves alternate; leaflets three, of a deep shining green; flowers axillary, in short racemes, of a pale greenish-white; berries whittish; seeds colourless, hard, or bony. Different species of this genus yield a viscid juice, which is highly poisonous, but at the same time very useful, as affording some of the most valuable varnishes,—particularly *R. vernix*, with which the Japanese varnish all their wooden utensils, as well as their doors and windows; and it is from this circumstance, and the best varnish being procured from that country, that we have the common term Japan, as expressing something varnished in a high degree.

All the species are possessed of such dangerous properties that they should be approached or handled with much caution, as many instances have occurred of serious inconvenience from merely taking a leaf into the hand. Loudon enumerates eighty-one species and ten varieties.

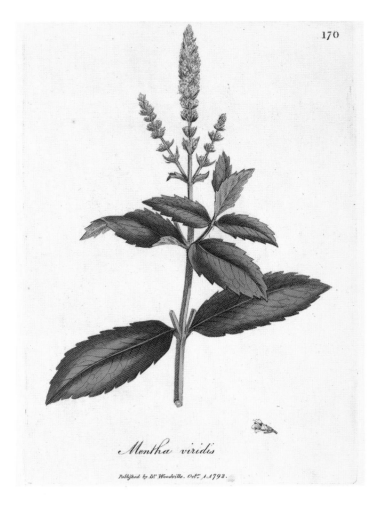

Mentha viridis

Published by Dr Woodville. Oct.r 1.1792.

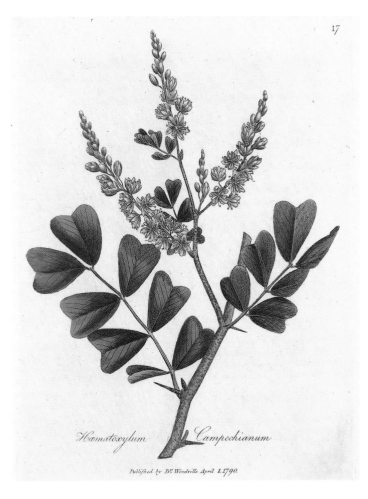

Hæmatoxylum Campechianum

Published by Dr Woodville April 1.1790.

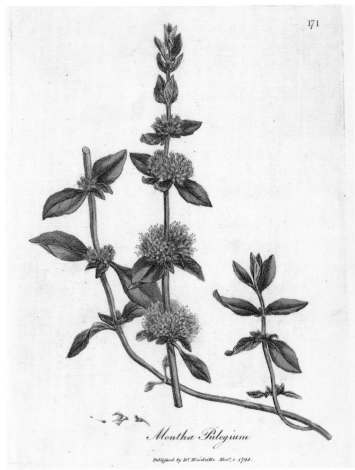

Mentha Pulegium

Published by Dr Woodville Nov.r 1.1792.

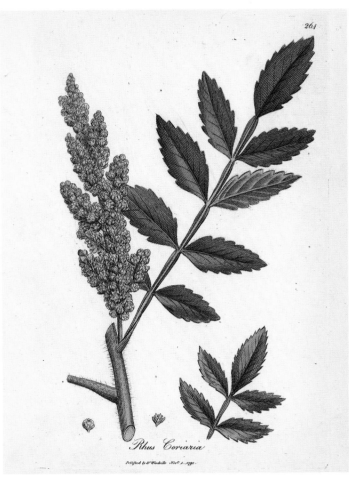

Rhus Coriaria

Published by Dr Woodville Nov.r 1.1791.

TOP LEFT: SPEARMINT, TOP RIGHT: LOGWOOD, BOTTOM LEFT: PENNY-ROYAL,
BOTTOM RIGHT: POISON-OAK

The *Rhus toxicodendron* is a virulent, acrid poison. The gas which it exhales while growing is sufficiently impregnated with its deleterious properties to cause in some particular constitutions very unpleasant, and even dangerous symptoms. "Calm relates, that of two sisters, one could manage the tree without being affected by its venom, whilst the other felt its exhalations as soon as she came within a yard of it, or even when she stood to leeward of it at a greater distance; that it had not the least effect upon him, though he made many experiments on it, and though the juice once squirted into his eye; but that, on another person's hand, which he covered very thick with it, the skin, in a few hours after, became as a piece of tanned leather, and peeled off afterwards in scales." According to Van Mons of Brussels, the gas which this plant exhales is carburetted hydrogen, holding a deleterious volatile principle. When examined during the day, this plant yields an innoxious watery fluid and nitrogen. It is only after sunset that the carburetted hydrogen and the deleterious principle are evolved. Dufresnoy introduced this remedy is cases of inveterate scabies and in epilepsy. He gave the extract in doses of from fifteen to twenty grains, two or three times a-day, with occasional success. Dr Brera gave the powdered leaves of the *R. radicans*, a much more virulent species, in doses of the fourteen part of a grain every four hours with marked success in paralysis. Dr Duncan tried the leaves of the *R. toxicodendron* in paralysis, but did not succeed in curing the disease. The medicine took effect so far as to cause pricking and tingling in the limbs of the patient.

YELLOW GENTIAN

Gentiana lutea

Class and Order, Pentandria Digynia. Nat. Ord. Gentianeæ.
Gen. Char. *Calix* four or five-cleft; *Corolla* sub-campanulate, funnel or salver-shaped, tubular at the base, destitute of nectariferous glands.

ALL the species of Gentian are intensely bitter. The present species is the one in common use,—its size rendering it more attainable than some other species. It is a native of Germany, Switzerland, and other parts of Europe, and thrives well in Britain. Roots perennial, penetrating deep into the earth, thick, fleshy; stems herbaceous, rising to three or more feet high, and having a profusion of thickly-clustered flowers, which grow in whorls, of a yellow colour; leaves large, boat-shaped, and deeply channelled. This is a handsome herbaceous plant, and merits a place in every garden. It is of easy cultivation, and bears transplanting and dividing better than some other kinds.

The various individuals composing the natural family of gentianæ are bitter, and febrifuge. The purest bitter I have met with is furnished by the *Gentiana chirayita*, which is used as a stomachick in the East Indies.

Gentian is one of the purest and best bitters in the pharmacopœia, and is useful in all cases where tonic bitters are indicated. In dyspepsia it is valuable either alone or combined with other bitters or with astringents, or aromatics. It raises the pulse, increases the appetite, and in some cases acts as an emmenagogue.

ALMOND

Amygdalus communis

Class and Order, Icosandria Monogynia. Nat. Ord. Rosaceæ.
Gen. Char. *Calix* of five segments, inferior; *Petals* five; *Drupe* containing a perforated nut.

THE tree producing the almond is highly ornamental, and well merits a place in all shrubberies and pleasure grounds; it forms a low tree, and early in the year produces a profusion of flowers. Both varieties, the *dulcis* and *amara*, are natives of Barbary, and the islands in the Mediterranean Sea, and are cultivated for the markets in the South of France, Italy, Spain, and the Levant. The best sweet or Jordan almonds are imported from Malaga, and the bitter ones from Mogadore. In France numerous varieties are cultivated; in England we rarely meet with any but the two above named, and the most beautiful variety, the double blossomed kind.

The kernel of the almond nut is demulcent, nutritive, and oleaginous. A bland fixed oil applicable to many domestic and pharmaceutic purposes is obtained from it by pressure. The bitter almond, which is only a variety of the sweet, contains a mucilaginous, albuminous solid matter, like the sweet almond, but it also yields with water a highly poisonous volatile oil,

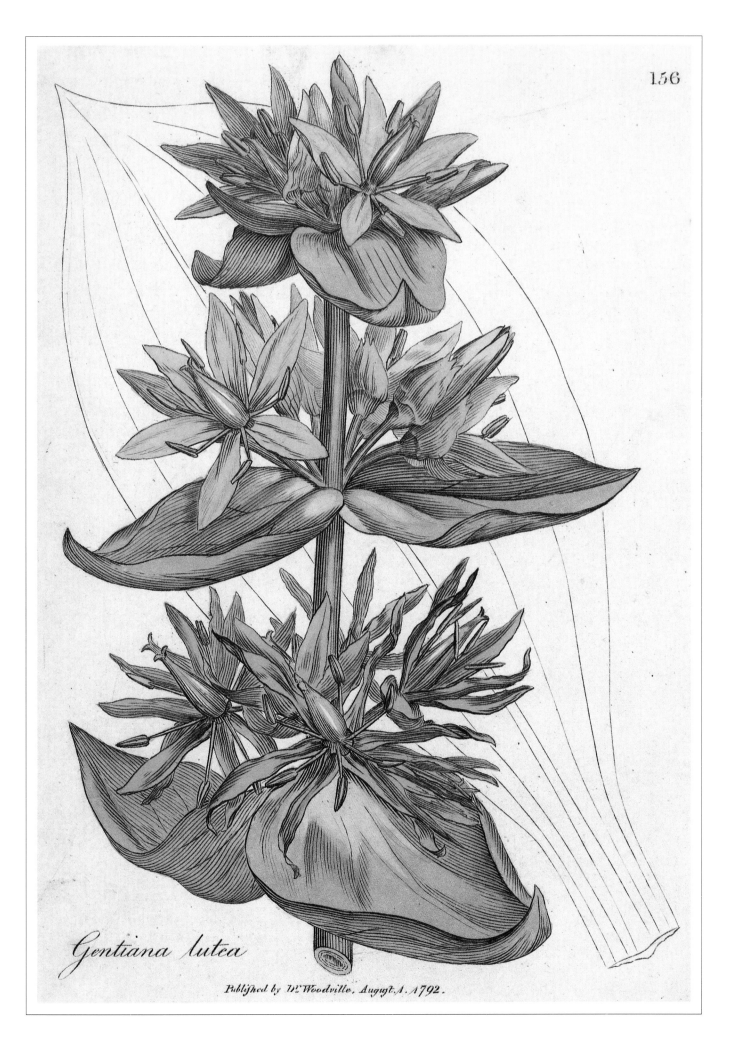

Gentiana lutea

Published by Dr. Woodville, August 1. 1792.

YELLOW GENTIAN

of a pleasant aromatic odour, and a warm biting taste. Its poisonous properties are owing to the presence of hydrocyanic acid, but the smell is quite independent of this acid, and belongs to the essential oil, which is not poisonous.

Many accidents have happened from custards and puddings beings too highly flavoured with the essential oil, and biscuits made with bitter almonds often produce unpleasant symptoms. The late Professor Gregory suffered an attack of urticaria, after eating any thing into which bitter almonds had been put.

OFFICIAL SQUILL

Scilla maritima

Class and Order, Hexandria Monogynia. Nat. Ord. Asphodeleæ.
Gen. Char. *Perianth* inferior, of six petaloid, spreading, deciduous leaves; *Filaments* fili-form, glabrous, inserted at the base of the perianth.

This species, which has been arranged by authors either in the genus *Scilla* or *Ornithogalum*, grows abundantly on the sandy hills of Spain and Portugal, and though occasionally found on the *shores* of France, Spain, Portugal, Italy, and the Mediterranean generally, yet, as remarked by Professor Link, in *Annals of Botany*, "the name of *maritima* is not quite proper, for the plant is seldom met with near the sea-shore, and sometimes very remote from it, as, for instance, at the foot of the Estrella mountains, which are at about one hundred miles from the sea."

Bulb large, tunicated, five or six inches in diameter, pear-shaped, from which in the month of May issues the flowering stem, in length from two to three feet, bearing at its extremity a long dense spike of dirty-white flowers, having a purple stripe along the under side; the leaves appear towards the close of summer, are a foot to eighteen inches long, pretty numerous, and generally waved at the edges. The bulbs are very tenacious of life; the late Dr Duncan showed me one which produced a flowering stem a year after it had been deposited in a case of the Materia Medica Museum, and the following year the same plant made a fresh attempt at vegetating, some leaves having made their appearance on the crown of the bulb; but it had not sufficient vigour to bring them to perfection. The most energetic of the recent bulbs are of a purple hue, which disappears if long kept; when wanted for use the whole of the exterior tunics that are dry should be removed as useless. The root is either dried whole, or cut into slices and dried, which is best done by artificial heat, as though the root loses the greater portion of its weight, what is evaporated appears to be an almost tasteless watery fluid. If exposed to the air after being dried it absorbs moisture, and soon becomes mouldy, and should be kept in closely-stopped bottles.

Squill is an excellent expectorant and diuretic when given in small doses; in large doses it acts as an emetic, and is apt to cause strangury. It is a general stimulant, and when combined with calomel acts chiefly on the kidneys. It is useful in chronic catarrh, asthma, and dropsy. Its taste is bitter and nauseous, and all the liquid preparations are more or less unpleasant. The most agreeable form in which it can be administered is that of pill. Squills owe their activity to a principle discovered by Vogel, *Scillitine*, but which he did not procure in a state of purity. Tilloy gives the following process for preparing it. He digests the dried root in strong alcohol, and evaporates the tincture thus formed to the consistence of syrup, then adds alcohol, sp. gr. 842; this leaves some extractive matter undissolved; he then pours off the alcoholic solution, and evaporates to the consistence of extract; and acts upon this with ether, which dissolves a fatty acid, and leaves the *Scillitine*, a grain of which is sufficient to kill a strong dog.

GAMBOGE

Garcinia cambogia

Class and Order, Dodecandria Monogynia. Nat. Ord. Guttiferæ.
Gen. Char. *Calix* four-leaved; *Petals* four; *Berry* eight-seeded, crowned by the peltate *Stigma*.

The above named plant is supposed to yield the gamboge of commerce, but the sources from whence the drug is obtained are so doubtful, that it is with some hesitation I particularize any as producing the official drug. By the British colleges the well-known pigment Gamboge or Camboge, is stated to be the production of *Stalagmites Cambogioides*, which is a native of the East Indies, and is said to grow in abundance on the banks of the river Kambogia, whence its

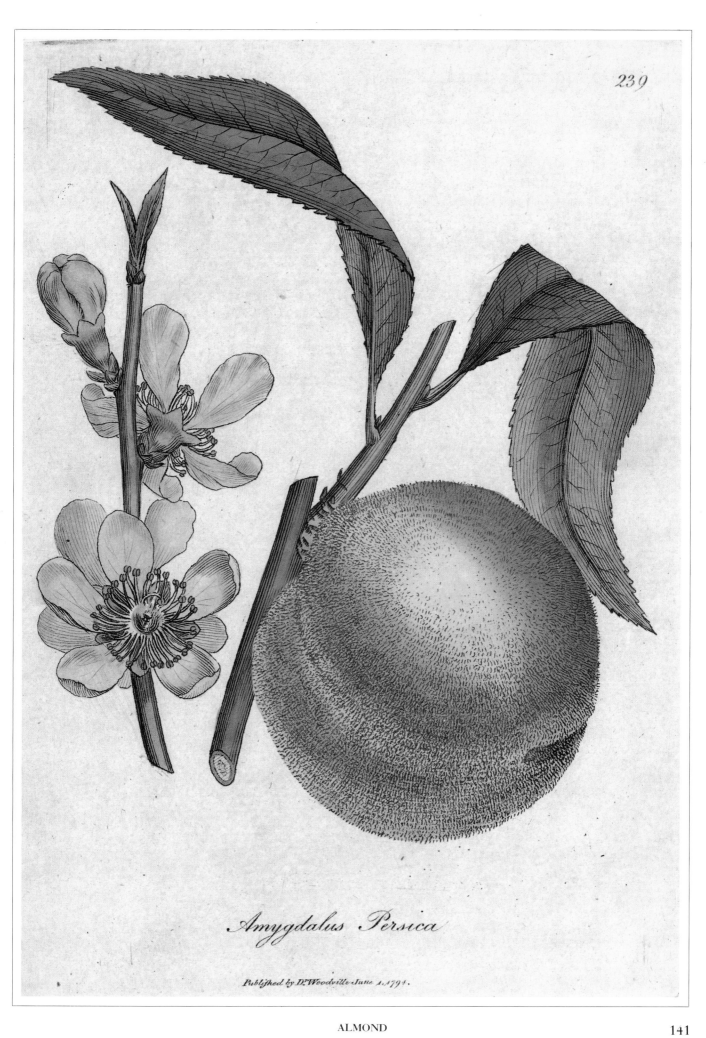

Amygdalus Persica

Published by Dr Woodville June 1, 1794.

ALMOND

name. A somewhat similar substance is obtained from the *Garcinia cambogia*, a tree found on the coast of Malabar; and a considerable variety of plants in the East Indies abound in a yellow fluid which hardens on exposure, and is indiscriminately known to druggists as Gamboge.

Numerous species yield a gamboge-like substance, and it may hereafter prove that many, if not most, plants whose natural juices are of the gamboge colour, are possessed of similar properties. Our native species which abound in this kind of juice are the *Glaucium luteum*, and *Chelidonium majus*, but I have not had an opportunity of examining either, for the purpose of ascertaining their qualities.

Gamboge when fine is of a dark yellow in mass, if moistened a bright yellow, and reduced to powder it is of a full golden yellow inclining to orange; it has a sickly unpleasant odour, and on handling adheres to the fingers; it is usually imported in rolls or flat cakes, and often contains seeds, leaves, pieces of stick, and other impurities.

Gamboge is a drastic purgative, and was long used as a vermifuge, particularly in tænia, but for the latter purpose it has yielded to oil of turpentine. It is still used occasionally, and acts well in cases of obstinate constipation.

GREAT ROUND-LEAVED SALLOW

Salix caprea

Class and Order, Diœcia Diandria. Nat. Ord. Salicineæ.
Gen. Char. Barren flower: *Scales* of the catkin single-flowered, imbricated, with a nectariferous gland at the base; *Perianth* wanting; *Stamens* one to five.
Fertile flower: *Scales* of the catkin single-flowered, imbricated, with a nectariferous gland; *Perianth* wanting; *Stigmas* two, often cleft; *Capsule* one-celled, two-valved, many-seeded; *Seeds* comose.

A very abundant species growing in hedges and dry banks. It has the largest leaves of any of our native species; is readily known by producing its large handsome blossoms before any of the leaves appear; it forms a moderate-sized tree, with spreading purplish slightly downy branches; in the Highlands, the bark is used for tanning leather, and the wood for a variety of agricultural purposes.

This is an intricate numerous family, the individuals of which frequently so nearly resemble each other, that it requires no small botanical acumen to distinguish the species. Loudon has one hundred and sixty-seven, besides varieties. All these agree in their qualities, varying only in the degree of astringency; the leaves and stems of all contain tannin; many produce galls of equal value with those of the oak.

Various species of willow are used in medicine. They all possess astringent, tonic, and febrifuge virtues, and have been proposed as substitutes for cinchona. They owe their activity to a proximate vegetable principle discovered by Leroux, and named by him *Salicine*. It is pretty extensively used in France as a tonic and febrifuge, and it was at one time held out as being equal to sulphate of quinine, but experience has not confirmed this statement.

COMMON BRITISH OAK

Quercus robur

Class and Order, Monœcia Polyandria. Nat. Ord. Cupuliferæ.
Gen. Char. Barren flower in a lax catkin or spike; *Perianth* single, five-cleft; *Stamens* five to ten.
Fertile flower: *Involucre* of many little scales, united into a cup; *Perianth* single, closely investing the germen, six-toothed; *Germen* three-celled; *Style* one; *Stigmas* three; *Nut* or *Acorn* one-celled, one-seeded, covered by the persistent, enlarged perianth, and surrounded at the base by the enlarged cup-shaped involucre.

The Oak is too well known to require description. The two species native of Britain, closely resemble each other,—differing little but in the comparative length of their fruit-stalks. The wood is hard and durable. It is of slow growth; prefers a deep strong soil, as its roots descend deep. Formerly its fruit afforded food for man, but is now rejected, and left for swine and other animals. Its bark is used for the purpose of the tanner, and the galls abounding on the petioles and leaves of several species are used for dyeing. The genus is principally confined to the temperate parts of the old and new continents. From the *Q. suber* is obtained cork, which is the exterior bark; this valuable article is stripped from the trees whilst standing, and, as another bark is beneath, the trees are not injured by the operation; the species is common to the more elevated parts of the south of Europe. Loudon names sixty-one species, and nearly the same number of varieties.

Oak-bark is a powerful astringent, and is useful in stopping internal hemorrhage, or profuse discharges of blood by the mouth and rectum. Its decoction and infusion are valuable gargles in relaxations of the throat and uvula, and it has been employed as an external application to thoracic aneurism. In the arts, oak-bark is used for tanning leather; it owes this property to the quantity of tannin or gallic acid which it contains.

COMMON LIQUORICE

Glycyrrhiza glabra

Class and Order, DIADELPHIA DECANDRIA. NAT. ORD. LEGUMINOSÆ.
Gen. Char. *Calix* bilabiate; *Upper lip* three-cleft, lower undivided; *Legume* ovate, compressed.

A hardy perennial herbaceous plant, a very old inhabitant of Britain's gardens, having been cultivated since 1562. Root long, often penetrating to the depth of four or five feet, and creeping to a considerable distance; stems, several from the same root, upright, striated, three feet or more high, with pinnated leaves; the pinnæ in six or eight pairs with a terminal one, which is on a longish footstalk; flowers in dense spikes; axillary, of a purple blue colour, diffusing when in blossom a very agreeable fragrance; legumes oblong, compressed, containing four to six kidney-shaped seeds.

The Liquorice has long been an object of cultivation for the sweet juice afforded by its roots. Pontefract in Yorkshire is celebrated for it, and the juice prepared in small flat pieces, is commonly known by the name of Pomfret cakes. It requires a light deep soil, and in land of this description I have known the soil dug out to the dept of four feet, at the bottom of which is laid a thick coat of cinder ashes, which prevents the root descending deeper. The sets or cuttings of the root are planted about four inches beneath the surface, and they reach the bottom of the trench by the end of the second year. As soon as they come in contact with the ashes they cease to elongate, and expand laterally, so that the roots are often an inch or more in diameter. The third year after planting, the roots are at perfection, and should be dug up soon after the stems are decayed, when they are succulent and fit for immediate use. The larger part of that grown in Britain is used by the porter-brewers as a substitute for malt, and to contribute to that flavour so much admired in London porter.

The stems in a young state are greedily devoured by cattle. There are several other species, one, *G. echinatus*, has been found in cultivation less saccharine and juicy than the present plant.

Liquorice root has an agreeable, sweet, mucilaginous taste; it is an excellent demulcent, and is said to have some expectorant qualities. It is not often prescribed in substance, and occasionally in the form of infusion or decoction. The extract, which is commonly known by the name of Liquorice, or black sugar, is not prepared by the apothecary, but is imported chiefly from Spain and Italy. It occurs in cylindrical rolls, which are usually covered with bay leaves. The decoction of the root, or the solution of the extract, are excellent vehicles for covering the taste of nauseous drugs, and are generaly palatable to children.

BITTER CUCUMBER, OR BITTER APPLE

Cucumis colocynthis

Class and Order, MONŒCIA MONADELPHIA. NAT. ORD. CUCURBITACEÆ.
Gen. Char. Male: *Calix* five-parted; *Corolla* of five petals; *Filaments* three.
Female: *Calix* five-parted; *Corolla* of five petals; *Pistil* three-cleft; *Seeds* with a sharp edge.

THIS species is abundant in Turkey, Nubia, various parts of Africa, and in Mediterranean islands. It is an annual plant, and requires the same culture as the melon and cucumber. The root is fibrous, and penetrates deep into the earth; stems slender, angular, branching, rough with coarse pellucid hairs, almost spines; leaves on long footstalks, deeply cut with an indefinite number of lobes; flowers small, axillary, solitary, of a yellow colour. The female flower resembles the male, and has filaments but not anthers. The fruit is round and smooth, of the size and colour of an orange, three-celled, each containing numerous ovate, compressed seeds, enveloped in a white spongy pulp.

The dried pulp is the part used in medicine; it is white, soft and porous, of an intensely bitter taste, but the seeds imbedded in it are nearly tasteless.

Colocynth is a powerfully drastic purgative, of an extremely bitter and nauseous taste. Its action is so violent, that it is seldom or never given uncombined. It frequently gives rise to tormina, and when taken in an overdose it acts as an acrid poison, and causes death by general peritonitis.

"A considerable number of severe cases of poisoning with this substance have occurred in the human subject; and a few have proved fatal. *Tulpius* notices the case of a man who was nearly carried off by profuse, bloody diarrhœa, in consequence of taking a decoction of three colocynth apples. *Orfila* relates that of a rag-picker, who, attemping to cure himself of a gonorrhœa by taking three ounces of colocynth, was seized with vomiting, acute pain in the stomach, profuse diarrhœa, dimness of sight, and slight delirium; but he recovered under the use of diluents and local blood-letting. In 1823 a coroner's inquest was held at London on the body of a woman who died in twenty-four hours with incessant vomiting and purging, in consequence of having swalled by mistake a teaspoonful and a-half of colocynth powder. *M. Carron d'Annecy* has communicated to Orfila the details of an instructive case, which also proved fatal. The subject was a locksmith, who took from a quack two glasses of decoction of colocynth to cure hemorrhoids, and was soon after attacked with colic, purging, heat in the belly, and dryness of the throat. Afterwards the belly became tense and excessively tender, and the stools were suppressed altogether. Next morning he had also retention of urine, retraction of the testicles and priapism. On the third day the retention ceased, but the other symtoms continued, and the skin became covered with clammy sweat, which preceded his death only a few hours. The intestines were red, studded with black spots, and matted together by fibrinous matter; the usual fluid of peritonitis was effused into the belly; the villous coat of the stomach was here and there ulcerated; and the liver, kidneys, and bladder also exhibited traces of inflammation."

KINO-TREE

Pterocarpus erinaceus

Class and Order, Nat. Ord. and Generic Character, See
P. santalinus.

THOUGH the present is considered the species producing the finest quality of the drug kino, the same, or a very similar substance, is afforded, not only by other species of the genus, but also by species belonging to different genera. The London College consider this species as producing kino, the Edinburgh College the *Eucalyptus resinifera,* and in the Dublin Pharmacopœia it is attributed to the *Butea frondosa.*

Each of these trees doubtless produce an analogous substance, resembling in appearance the true kino, and possessed of similar properties, as do a variety of others. Their concrete juices are of a deep-red colour, powerfully astringent, and vary, the one from the other, in their greater or less brilliancy of colour.

The present is a low tree, with a tortuous stem, covered with ash-coloured bark; leaves deciduous; flowers numerous, yellow, on short curved pedicels, with a pair of small lanceolate bracteas at the base of each; fruit a compressed orbicular pod, with a leaf-like margin, containing a single kidney-shaped seed. It is a native of Senegal, from whence specimens were transmitted to Europe by the enterprising Mungo Park. The drug is procured by wounding the tree.

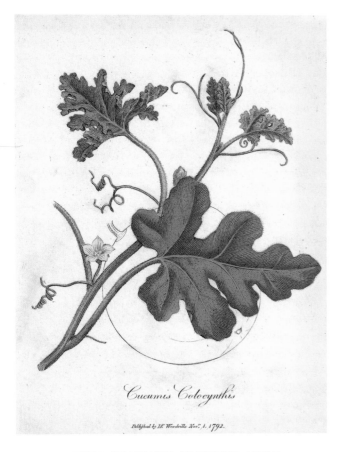

Cucumis Colocynthis

Published by Dr Woodville Nov.ʳ 1. 1792.

BITTER-CUCUMBER OR BITTER-APPLE

"The juice is at first very fluid and pale-coloured, but, as it concretes, becomes of a deep blood-red, and is finally so brittle that its collection is attended with some difficulty."

A good deal of discrepancy of opinion exists as to the sources from which kino is procured. "The kino," says Dr Thomson, "originally introduced into the pale of the Materia Medica of the British colleges, came from Africa; and, from a specimen sent home by Mungo Park, it has been ascertained to be the juice of a species of Pterocarpus, which Decandolle has described in the Encyclopédie Methodique under the specific name *Erinacea*. The London College, overlooking the fact, that scarcely any of this kind of kino is now found in the market, has designated this plant in their pharmacopœia as the only source of kino. The Edinburgh College has put down kino as the production of the *Eucalyptus reinifera*, a tree which is a native of New Holland and Van Dieman's land, belonging to the natural order Myrtaceæ. The greater part of the kino now found in commerce is the inspissated juice of the *Nauclea gambir*, a plant which is a native of India, and belonging to the natural order Rubiaceæ." Kino is a very powerful astringent, and is, like others of its class, useful in hemorrhage and profuse diarrhœa. It has been recommended, in union with opium, in pyrosis. Dr Thomson proposes, or rather hints, at its probable use in gleet.

OFFICINAL OR PALMATED RHUBARB

Rheum palmatum

Class and Order, ENNEANDRIA TRIGYNIA. NAT. ORD. POLYGONEÆ.
Gen. Char. *Corolla* six-cleft, persistent; *Seed* one, three-sided.

A HARDY herbaceous perennial, growing freely in most soils and situations, a native of various parts of Russia, but generally cultivated over Europe. The roots of the different species appear to possess similar properties, and it is a matter of doubt from which species the officinal drug is obtained. In Britain the roots grow to a large size, and many persons dry and use them for the same purposes as the imported drug. They should be dug up when the leaves are decayed, thoroughly cleared from earth, and the decaying parts of the leaves and stems removed; the roots should be cut into pieces, and carefully dried, either by exposure to the air, or by moderate heat. I have frequently prepared roots of this species, as also those of *R. undulatum*, which could not be detected from the finest foreign samples by several eminent apothecaries.

Several species are now largely cultivated for their leaf-stalks, which are used for domestic purposes as substitutes for unripe gooseberries; the plant may be blanched in the manner of sea-kale, when the whole of it, excepting the root, is fit for the table.

Rhubarb is a valuable tonic purgative; its action is usually mild, and requires to be assisted by some other purgative, such as aloes or calomel. The root, in its entire state, is a favourite remedy with those whose bowels are habitually constipated, and who lead a sedentary life. They chew a small portion of it every morning; and the taste, though are first disagreeable, becomes by habit less so, till, at last, as I have been assured, it becomes rather pleasant than otherwise. It has been recommended as a vermifuge, but its action in this way is not remarkable. In the diseases of children it is a very safe remedy, as it seldom acts too violently. When toasted, it loses nearly the whole of its purgative properties and becomes an excellent tonic. The late Dr Duncan frequently prescribed it when thus prepared.

GRAPE VINE

Vitis vinifera

Class and Order, PENTANDRIA MONOGYNIA. NAT. ORD. VINIFERÆ.
Gen. Char. *Calix* five-cleft; *Petals* cohering at the apex, deciduous; *Berry* five-seeded.

THIS well known plant is supposed to be a native of Greece; but, from its having so long been an object of culture, its native country, like that of wheat, is by no means satisfactorily ascertained. In all civilized countries, whose temperature allow of its cultivation, the vine stands conspicuous among fruit trees. It was formerly extensively grown in many parts of England in large plantations, or vineyards, as it is now on the continent of Europe, but for the last two centuries, it has gradually declined, and at this time vineyards are unknown in Britain.

The vine is too well known to require description. In other countries its varieties for the desert or manufacture of wine are numerous, but the finest kinds for the table are said to be raised in Britain. In Scotland it rarely matures its fruit in the open ground; but in the hot summer of 1826, grapes were generally ripened; and, in favourable situation, they were so last autumn in various parts. Though capable of enduring the British winter in the open ground, grapes are more generally grown in houses erected for the purpose; and, with the care which British cultivators bestow upon them, attain a superiority in size and flavour, that, in other countries, under more favourable circumstances of climate, they do not attain to.

The Grape vine appears to be confined to the old world, as, though now cultivated in America, the only native species is the Fox-grape, *Vitis vulpina*, the fruit of which, from its peculiar flavour, cannot enter into competition with the true grapes. Fifteen species are enumerated, but it is probable that several of these are only varieties. The vine attains to a great age, vineyards being now in bearing that were planted at the end of the fifteenth century.

The fruit of the vine is more an article of diet than medicine. When dried they become what are called raisins. In this state they are laxative and mucilaginous, but not so cooling as the recent fruit.

Wine is the juice of the grape altered by fermentation. The numerous varieties depend both upon the quantity of sugar in the must, and on the mode of fermentation. The intoxicating property depends on the quantity of alcohol which it contains. Sherry is that which is commonly used in medicine. Port is generally given in fever, and is more tonic and restorative.

OFFICINAL GUAIACUM, OR LIGNUM VITÆ-TREE

Guaiacum officinale

Class and Order, DECANDRIA MONOGYNIA. NAT. ORD. ZYGOPHYLLEÆ.

Gen. Char. *Calix* of five unequal parts; *Petals* five, equal; *Capsule* angular, two to five-celled.

THIS species forms a tree of considerable magnitude, attaining the height of forty or fifty feet, and from four to five feet in circumference. It is of slow growth. Its roots strike deep into the soil, in which respect it differs from the generality of timber in hot climates, which usually spread their roots horizontally and near the surface; leaves abruptly pinnate; flowers pale-blue, which are succeeded by roundish compressed berries.

The Guaiac is valuable as a timber tree,—the wood is hard, durable, but very heavy, and is much used by turners, also for ships' blocks. Every part of the tree possesses medicinal qualities, but it is the wood and an exudation from it that are in general use. This substance, which spontaneously exudes, contains the active medicinal properties, and is much to be preferred to that procured by artificial means. It is collected in the form of tears. This gum-resin is also obtained by placing billets of the wood, bored longitudinally, across the fire; the resinous matter is melted, runs into the cavity, and is collected at the extremity; in this state, though a powerful medicine, it is less valuable than when naturally formed. It has held its reputation for upwards of three centuries, and was introduced into Europe by the Spaniards in the year 1508.

Guaiac acts on the animal economy as a general stimulus. It is useful in the sequelæ of syphilis, and in scrofulous affections; it is also prescribed in gout; the resin acts in the same way as the wood, but is more powerful. It acts as a diaphoretic if the patient be kept warm, and as a diuretic if he be freely exposed to cold air. The changes of colour which guaiac resin undergoes are remarkable.

SOCOTRINE ALOE

Aloe socotrina

Class and Order, HEXANDRIA MONOGYNIA. NAT. ORD. ASPHODELEÆ.

Gen. Char. *Flower* tubular, monopetalous, six-cleft, secreting honey at its base; *Filaments* inserted into the receptacle; *Capsule* three-celled, three-valved, many-seeded; *Seeds* in two rows, with a membranous edge.

MUCH uncertainty prevails respecting the species from which the finest kinds of this drug are obtained; that introduced from the island of Socotora, and named *socotrina*, is considered as yielding the best sort. It is of a deep bright brown when in mass, but small pieces when viewed between the eye and the light appear of a

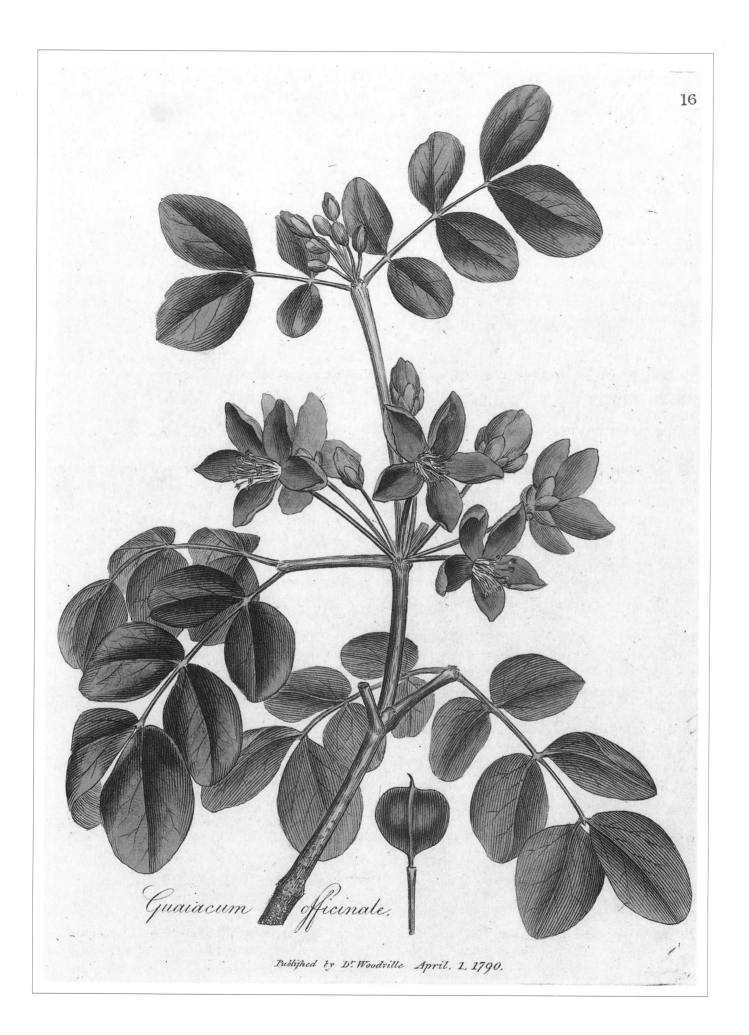

Guaiacum officinale.

Published by Dr Woodville April. 1. 1790.

GUAIACUM OR LIGNUM VITAE TREE

full reddish-yellow, perfectly clear and free from impurities.

All the species of aloe are of curious structure, they vary exceedingly in form, yet always retain sufficient of their essential characters to enable any one who has once seen an *aloe* to recognize them. In their native countries some kinds acquire an altitude and size that entitle them to be called trees, whilst others are so diminutive that a common wine-glass would contain several flowering plants; they all secrete large quantities of delicious honey; which in many kinds is constantly distilling from the flowers. They are succulent, of easy culture, and require to be kept in the stove during the greater part of the year, and to be sparingly supplied with water; the species are numerous, ninety-six being described in Loudon's Encyclopædia of Plants.

Three kinds of aloes occur in commerce. The Socotrine, the hepatic or Barbadoes, and the Caballine. Of the two first the Socotrine is the most valued, but not a few practitioners in Britain prefer the hepatic, which acts more effectually, and is less subject to adulteration. Aloes act chiefly on the colon and rectum, and are therefore improper in hæmorrhoids and in pregnancy. They are usually combined with some other purgative, such as rhubarb, colocynth, sulphate of potass, soap, or with some saline substance. When a habitual purgative is required, aloes in combination is one of the best we can employ, as the dose rarely requires to be increased, as that of almost all other purgatives does when long continued. In obstruction of the menstrual and hæmorrhoidal discharges, aloes are useful.

Braconnot found a peculiar substance in all the varieties of aloes, to which he has given the name of bitter of aloes. The Socotrine and Barbadoes are the kinds used in medicine; the Caballine is only used in veterinary surgery.

WHITE, OR OPIUM POPPY

Papaver somniferum

Class and Order, Nat. Ord. and Gen. Character, see *P. Rhœas.*

Root annual; leaves and stems glaucous; flowers usually white, sometimes with a purple eye, and varying through every shade of purple and scarlet, and with single or double flowers. This is one of the most shewy of Britain's annuals, is universally cultivated in gardens, and is to be found growing wild in the vicinity of large towns and on the banks of streams.

All the species of poppy yield the well-known drug opium, but this species produces it in the greatest abundance and of superior quality; it is yielded by the garden varieties equally with the common kind; when cultivated for medicinal purposes, it should be sown on a light rich soil, and be constantly supplied with water until the capsules are half grown, at which time the waterings must be discontinued; the capsules should be cut across the rind without penetrating to the seeds, in the evening; during the night a considerable quantity of juice exudes from the wound, which should be carefully collected the following morning, and this operation be continued as long as any of the opium flows; the juice as obtained should be carefully kneaded together, and be exposed to the air and sun to allow evaporation freely; when the mass has hardened, it should be no longer exposed, but, after being enveloped in some of the leaves, should be kept from the air.

Like all narcotics, opium exerts in the first instance a stimulant action, and the duration of this depends entirely on the quantity given. If a large dose be taken, the stimulant effects are not marked, and we only see the narcotic or depressing effects. If the dose be small then the stimulant properties manifest themselves, and the narcotic qualities either show themselves slightly or not at all. If the dose be repeated before the excitement is over, then the narcotism is put off, and it is thus that opium-eaters keep up that mental excitement which at last proves so injurious. Opium has been said to excite the mental powers, while alcohol or wine acts more immediately on the animal, but this is not by any means ascertained, as the Turks use it as an Aphrodisiac, and to inspire them with courage. When taken habitually in large doses, opium produces the most baneful effects. The powers of body and mind become worn out; melancholy of the deepest nature supervenes, unless when the person is under the influence of the drug. The action of opium on the system is much influenced by sex, temperature, age, climate, and custom. Women are more easily affected by opium than men, and nausea more frequently follows a full dose; young people are more readily stimulated than old; sanguine temperaments are also more readily excited by this stimulus than melancholic, and nervous than lymphatic. Climate so far influences the action of opium, that a smaller dose acts more effectually in a warm than in a cold climate. Custom has a most powerful influence on the action of opium; for we know that men have brought themselves to take three or four drachms of opium daily, and that a drachm a day is not an uncommon dose for an opium-eater. Opium is the most valuable narcotic we possess; it is capable of being combined with so many other medicines; and its effects are so much under the control of the physician. It is antispasmodic and astringent, and its anodyne properties are remarkable. When combined with a diaphoretic, opium increases its powers, but does not lose its own; it moderates the violence of a cathartic; diminishes the irritation which many expectorants otherwise cause; retains by its astringent properties many remedies which would otherwise pass out of the system; allays external inflammation, and gives relief in rheumatic pains. In short, we may say, that, in the hands of a judicious practitioner, opium almost entirely supersedes the use of other narcotics where there is no consitutional peculiarity which prevents the exhibition of it.

The chemical history of opium is extremely interesting, from the complexity of its composition. Sertuerner, an apothecary in Eimbech, discovered its active principle, *morphia*, in 1803, but it did not attract general attention till 1817.

Four other crystalline substances have been lately discovered in opium, *Narceine* by Pelletier, *Meconine* by Couerbe, *Codein* by Robiquet, and *para-morphine*. The *narceine* and *meconine* have hitherto been procured in very small quantity, and have not yet been applied to any useful purpose. Codein was discovered by Robiquet in the washings of the morphia precipitated from the muriate. It is prepared by evaporating the washings with a slight excess of muriatic acid till they form crystals on cooling; these are acted upon with caustic potass, which dissolves the morphia and combines with the muriatic acid, while the codein is left. It is purified by repeated crystallization in alcohol, water, or ether, or by being united with an acid and precipitated by an alkali. Para-morphine is not

much known as yet, and does not promise to be of much interest. I found that opium yielded an empyreumatic oil virulently poisonous, and which no doubt is the cause of the intoxication which the smoke of opium produces in the Turks, Chinese, and other Eastern nations who use it in that form.

Since the discovery of morphia, it has always been considered as the active principle of opium, and though it may not be quite so powerful as the proportional quantity of opium, yet we must still consider it in that light. The muriate of morphia is now very extensively used instead of laudanum, and agrees with constitutions where laudanum never could be taken from the disagreeable effects to which it gave rise. I have tried muriate of morphia in cholera, and found it superior to laudanum or solid opium, as it did not seem to cause determination to the head, which all preparations of opium itself seemed to do.

Codein is crystalline, transparent, and colourless; its taste is bitter, and similar to morphia; when the nitrate or muriate of Codein is taken in a dose of six grains, it causes general excitement, followed by languor, and accompanied by a sense of pricking or itching, chiefly about the neck and hands. It seems that the disagreeable itching produced by muriate of morphia, and other preparations of opium, is to be referred to this substance. Among seven or eight gentlemen who took this substance, as prepared by Dr Gregory, all were excited, and the excitement was chiefly intellectual; all were depressed after its stimulant action had gone off, and two in such an alarming degree as to be obliged to take stimuli of various kinds. The itching took place in all, but in some less than others; I hardly felt it at all, and was less affected by its exciting or depressing effects that any of the others who tried it. Dr Gregory states, that the muriate of morphia when freed from codein, of which it contains a considerable per centage, acts with even less chance of causing the disagreeable effects of opium. Meconic acid is of no use in medicine; it is a solid crystalline substance of an austere, bitter, sour taste.

The preparations of opium for internal use are numerous, but do not now call for so much attention, since the salts of morphia have become so common and so cheap. The "black drop," Battley's sedative liquor, are supposed to be citrates and tartrates of morphis, and are superior to laudanum. The ammoniated tincture of opium is an excellent preparation, and very useful in pectoral affections; it is known by the name of "Scotch paregoric elixir." The camphorated tincture is another very good preparation in pectoral complaints, and is known by the name of "English paregoric."

I shall quote Dr Christison's remarks on opium as a poison, and on the means of detecting it after death, as there is no other work which gives so full an account, and at the same time so succinct and minute a detail.

"To the medical jurist opium is one of the most important of poisons; since there is hardly any other whose effects come more frequently under his cognizance. It is the poison most generally resorted to by the timid to accomplish self-destruction, for which purpose it is peculiarly well adapted on account of the gentleness of its operation. It has also been often the source of fatal accidents, which naturally arise from its extensive employment in medicine. It has likewise been long very improperly employed to create amusement. And in recent times it has been made use of to commit murder, and to induce stupor previous to the commission of robbery. *Mr Burnett*, in his work on Criminal Law, has mentioned a trial for murder in 1800, in which the prisoners were accused of having committed the crime by poisoning with opium; and although a verdict of *not proven* was returned, there is little doubt that the deceased, an adult, was poisoned in the way supposed. A few years ago a very remarkable trial took place at Paris, where poisoning was alleged to have been affected by means of the alkaloid principle of opium; and the prisoner, a young physician of the name of Castaing, was condemned and executed."

STRONG-SCENTED OR POISON LETTUCE

Lactuca virosa

Class and Order, Syngenesia Æqualis. Nat. Ord. Compositæ.
Gen. Char. *Involucre* imbricated, cylindrical, its scales with a membranous margin; *Receptacle* naked; *Pappus* simple, stipitate.

The *Lactuca virosa* is occasionally met with in various parts of Britain, but is not a common plant; it usually grows on dry chalky soils. It flowers in July and August, and the seeding plants, appear towards the end of September. They do not always flower the following year, but produce a clustre of leaves which spread in a circular form; but, as the plant approaches to flowering, the greater part of the radical leaves die away, and the stems have only a few distantly placed leaves; flowers small, pale yellow; these do not expand except in fine sunny weather, but the seed is perfected whether the flowers expand or not. The whole plant abounds in a milky juice, possessing narcotic properties of a similar nature with those of opium, and without its constipating quality; the juice is collected in a similar way to opium, and is obtained from the plants by nipping off the extremities of the branches from which the juice exudes.

Dr Duncan Senior was the first who called the attention of the profession to the Garden Lettuce as a medicine, and by him the concrete juice was introduced under the name of Lactucarium. But the drug now prepared is obtained from *L. virosa*. It is anodyne and soporific, and agrees with most people even where morphia is followed by unpleasant effects. The sleep which Lactucarium causes is calm and refreshing, and is seldom disturbed by unpleasant dreams. An extract one-half the strength of Lactucarium, and prepared at one-sixth the price, can be obtained by boiling the flowers, stem, and leaves, when they begin to wither, in water for some hours, and then evaporating. The Lactucarium prepared by Messrs Duncan and Flockhart of this country is the finest and best which can be met with, and is of uniform strength. A great number of the continental chemists have analyzed the substance, for the purpose of procuring morphia, but they have been disappointed. I tried it also, and neither obtained morphia nor any other substance at all resembling it. Its empyreumatic oil is somewhat similar in appearance to that of opium.

BLACK HELLEBORE OR CHRISTMAS ROSE

Helleborus niger

Class and Order, Nat. Ord. and Generic Character, see *H. fœtidus*.

This species acquires its specific name from the

Pl 44

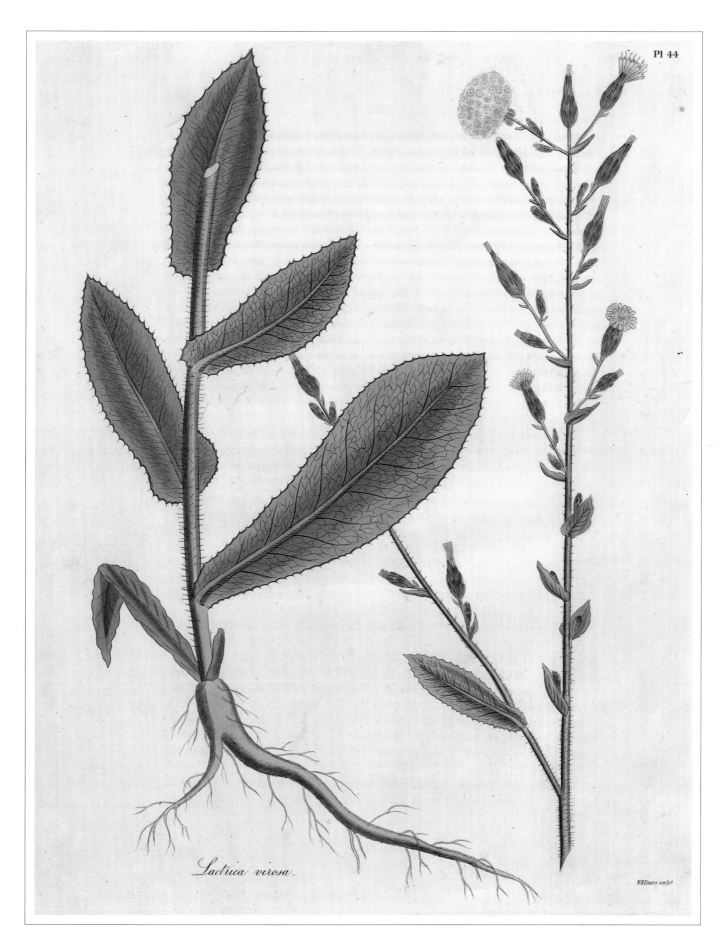

Lactuca virosa.

W.Elinars sculpt

STRONG-SCENTED OR POISON LETTUCE

black colour of its roots; it is a hardy perennial; flowering from the end of December to the middle of March, or later; and, from its usually producing its flowers during the winter, has acquired its common appellation of Christmas Rose.

Root knotty; externally blackish; within white; producing numerous fibres that descend deep into the soil; leaves growing on long footstalks immediately from the root, of a deep shining green, and deeply divided into five or more segments; flowers large, mostly solitary; at first white, but changing to a pale red, and finally a dusky purple, produced on scapes arising directly from the root. The Black Hellebore is a native of Austria, Italy, and other parts of Europe, bears climate exceedingly well, and is well worth a place in every garden, as it is not apt to encroach upon its neighbours, and produces its flower at a season when but few others can compete with it.

The *Helleborus niger* is purgative and emetic when given in a full dose, and emmenagogue and diuretic when prescribed in small quantity. It does not possess any advantage over jalap, scammony, or any brisk stimulating purgative; and, as it is poisonous, it ought never to be used for its purgative properties alone. It is said to be useful in small doses as a stimulating diuretic.

NUX VOMICA OR POISON-NUT

Strychnos nux vomica

Class and Order, Pentandria Monogynia. Nat. Ord. Apocyneæ.
Gen. Char. *Corolla* tubular, five-cleft; *Berry* one-celled, with a woody rind; *Seeds* two to five.

This plant is common on the coast of Coromandel and other parts of the East Indies. It forms a low tree with a crooked stem, and smooth ash-coloured bark; leaves nearly round, smooth, shining, entire; fruit a berry the size of an orange, and of a similar colour; the rind woody, filled with a colourless pulp, in which the seeds or nuts are imbedded; seeds flat and round, about as large as a shilling, and full a quarter of an inch thick; covered with fine silky hairs.

Apocyneæ, to which this genus belongs, is composed of a numerous tribe of plants, all of suspicious nature, and though a few possess innoxious properties, the larger part are active poisons. The seeds of the *Cerbera tanghin* are of so deadly a nature that a single one is sufficient to destroy twenty persons. Those of St Ignatius Bean, and a variety of others of this family, are well known poisons, but the bark of *Strychnos pseudo-quina* is said to be fully equal to Cinchona in the cure of intermittent fevers, and even the pulp contained in the fruit of the present plant may be eaten without inconvenience.

Nux vomica is an active and virulent poison, and is sometimes used as an instrument of self-destruction, and even as a means of committing murder, though, from its extremely bitter taste, it could not be easily given without the person's knowledge. The effects of this poison on man and animals are very violent; pain and heat in the stomach, constriction of the gullet, twitchings in the limbs, spasmodic action of the diaphragm, unsteady walk, giddiness and nausea are the first symptoms; these are succeeded by violent spasms, convulsive action of the limbs, and opisthotonos and tetanus. Convulsion follows convulsion, and death ensues at a period more or less distant from the time at which the dose was taken, according to the quantity swallowed. Dr Christison mentions numerous fatal cases, and also some where recovery took place, and others where death did not occur from the primary effects of the poison, but from inflammation of the stomach and intestines. Strychnia was discovered in the year 1818 by Pelletier and Caventou in the Nux vomica and in the Faba St Ignatii, and more recently in the Tieuté or Upas poison of Java, and the Urari of Guiana. Notwithstanding its poisonous qualities, it is used in medicine, and, whether given in the form of nux vomica, or in its purer form of strychnia, it acts very beneficially in some kinds of paralysis, in amaurosis, and other diseases where the nervous system is the seat of the disease. When given in the form of powder, nux vomica ought to be prescribed in a very small dose at first; two or at most three grains will be found sufficient. When strychnia is used, it ought to be combined with an acid, and about the sixteenth of a grain given at first. When violent twitchings of the limbs are observed, or when constitutional disturbance is caused, the medicine ought to be immediately stopped.

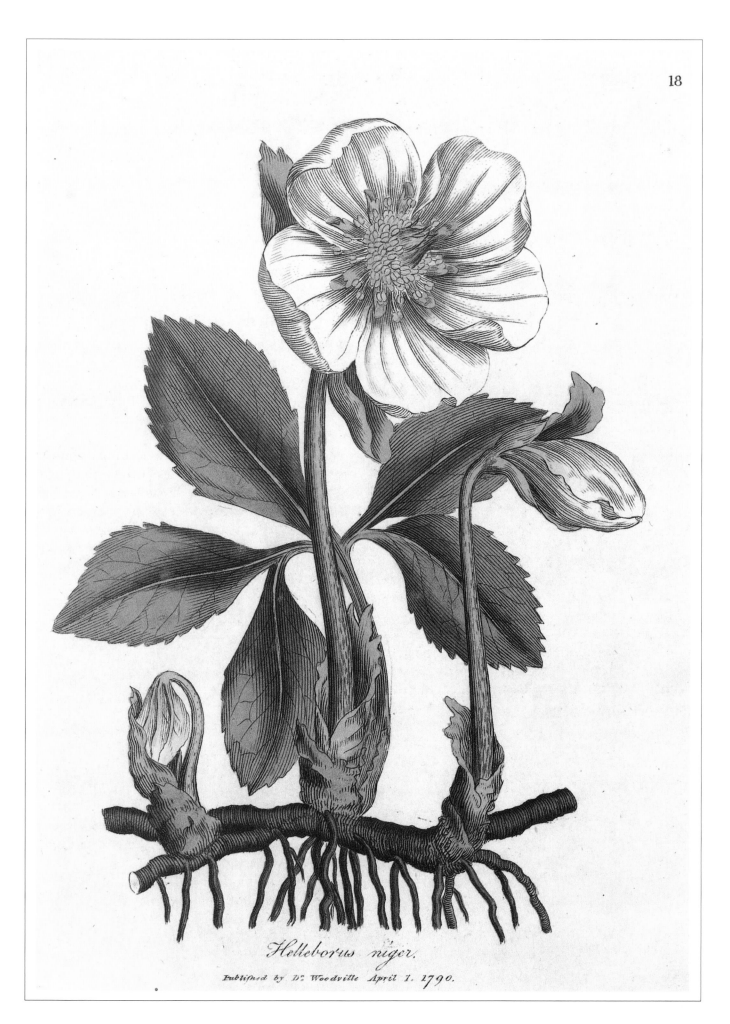

Helleborus niger.

Published by Dʳ. Woodville April 1. 1790.

BLACK HELLEBORE OR CHRISTMAS ROSE

SIMAROUBA

Simarouba officinalis

**Class and Order, DECANDRIA MONOGYNIA. NAT. ORD.
SIMARUBACEÆ.**
Gen. Char. *Calix* small, five-parted; *Petals* five; *Stem*
with a scale at the base; *Style* cleft.

———————

IT forms a tall tree, with smooth gray bark
blotched with yellow; the leaves are pinnate;
flower monœcious, pale yellow; male and female
flower growing on the same panicles; the fruit
consists of five smooth, ovate, purple-black,
one-celled berries on a common receptacle,
which open spontaneously when ripe; they bear
some resemblance to damsons in shape and
colour, from whence they have obtained the
provincial application of Mountain Damson.

This species with the *excelsa* were removed
from the genus *Quassia* by Decandolle, who
retains only the *Quassia amara* in that genus,
which he distinguishes from the present one by
its possessing hermaphrodite flowers, whilst the
Simarouba bears male and female flowers on the
same stem, or is polygamous. The officinal part
is the bark of the root, which is of an intensely
bitter taste, and is imported into Britain from
the West Indies, where it is a native, as well as
several parts of South America.

The bark of the root of the *Simarouba officinalis* is fibrous, rough, covered with warts, and
scaly; it is imported in large pieces; it has very
little smell, and a pure bitter taste. Where a
simple bitter is required it is useful, and can be
given in fevers and imflammatory diseases, as it
does not accelerate the pulse or produce those
constitutionally stimulant effects which almost
all other tonics do. It has been much recommended in anorexia, chronic diarrhœa, and
dyspepsia.

LOFTY OR ASH-LEAVED
SIMAROUBA

Simarouba excelsa

Class and Order, Nat. Ord. and Generic Character, see
S. officinalis.

———————

THIS, like the preceding species, forms a tall tree,
and is also a native of the West Indies. It often
attains to the height of one hundred feet. Leaves

pinnate; leaflets opposite, on petiols, smooth,
entire, pointed, with a terminal one; flowers in
large clusters, of a pale yellowish-green; fruit is
the size of a large currant, of a deep purple
black. The whole of the plant is of an intensely
bitter taste, more so than the preceding, and the
wood is imported in thick billets, which are
reduced to chips or shavings for the purpose of
the druggist. The two species now named, as
well as the *Quassia amara*, are frequently used
by brewers as substitutes for hops; they are said
to afford the purest vegetable bitters.

The *Quassia amara* is a low shrub with long
spikes of a pale but bright scarlet colour, these
are hermaphrodite; leaves pinnate, leaflets
opposite, in two pairs, and a terminal one,
connected one to the other by their winged
foot-stalks; there is no apparent resemblance
between this and the *Simaroubas*.

The wood of the Quassia, or *Sinarouba excelsa*, is the part used in medicine; it is said by
some to be that of the root, by others to be that
of the tree itself; its bitterness is more intense
than the preceding species, and it is much more
frequently prescribed. Dr Duncan supposes it to
have narcotic powers. It is sometimes
fraudulently substituted for hops by brewers,
though a very heavy penalty is incurred by such
a proceeding.

BALSAM OF COPAIVA OR
COPAIBA

Copaifera officinalis

**Class and Order, DECANDRIA MONOGYNIA. NAT. ORD.
LEGUMINOSÆ.**
Gen. Char. *Calix* wanting; *Petals* four; *Pod* one-seeded.

———————

THE tree producing the Copaiva Balsam is a
native of various parts of South America, is of
lofty growth, and forms a large branching head;
stems covered with ash-coloured bark; leaves
pinnate; flowers in long lax spikes. The drug is
obtained by boring the tree to the pith, near the
base of the trunk, when it flows abundantly, in
the form of a clear colourless liquid, which is
thickened, and acquires a yellowish colour by
age. The operation is performed two or three
times in the same year; and from the older trees
the best balsam is obtained.

Copaiba is used as an expectorant in chronic

catarrh, it is powerfully diuretic, and in moderate doses excites the natural functions of the kidneys, and increases the secretion of urine; in over-doses it inflames the kidneys; and it should never be administered when any tendency to ulceration is evidenced in these organs; it may be given either in a fluid state, or formed into soap by combining it with an alkali, by which its active properties are not diminished. The essential oil of copaiva is rising in estimation, and is freqently administered in cases where the balsam would be objectionable.

In a fluid state it may be given in doses from gr.xxx. to 1oz, combined with sugar and any bland fluid; the dose of soap is from twelve grains to a scruple. From its powerful effects on the urinary organs, it is successfully employed in the chronic states of gonorrhœa and gleet and for fluor albus.

TRAGACANTH PLANTS

Astragalus. Species various

Class and Order, Diadelphia Decandria. Nat. Ord. Leguminosæ.
Gen. Char. *Keel* of the *Corolla* obtuse; *Legume* two-celled, (more or less perfectly;) *Cells* formed by the inflexed margins of the lower suture.

Gum Tragacanth appears to be the produce of a variety of species belonging to the extensive genus *Astragalus*, and, not as generally esteemed, of an individual species. It is probable that this gum, if not common to the whole genus, is so to that section of it whose petioles are persistent, and which, after the fall of the leaves, become indurated and spinous. The species that produce the officinal drug are natives of Persia. The greater number of the species are small prostrate plants of but a few inches in height; a few attain to that of two feet; but they are all of straggling growth.

The drug is usually in vermiform, crooked, thread-like masses, of a pearly white colour, semitransparent, brittle, insipid, and without odour. Tragacanth differs very much from gum-Arabic in its properties. From its greater viscidity, it is employed in the manufacture of troches; otherwise gum-Arabic is preferred, in most cases, as it is simply useful as a demulcent.

GUM GALBANUM

Galbanum officinale

Class and Order, Pentandria Digynia. Nat. Ord. Umbelliferæ.

So little information is at present obtained of the plant producing the Gum Galbanum, that I shall only remark, it is certainly not procured from *Bubon galbanum* of Linnæus. From seeds found among the gum, Mr D. Don considers the plant belongs to a new genus, for which he proposes the name of Galbanum. This, as well as the plants producing Assafœtida and Ammoniacum, are probably natives of Persia, and the drug is imported into Britain from India and the Levant.

Galbanum is imported in masses, also in tears; it is of pale yellowish colour; the tears of which the larger masses are composed are clear, of a whitish hue, of a bitter taste, and a strong unpleasant odour, but without the alliaceous smell of Assafœtida. It abounds in impurities, such as leaves, sticks, seeds, and often sand; when of good quality it is brittle, and is without any other impurities than portions of the stems, leaves, and seeds; is rendered brittle by cold, and readily softens by heat; such samples as abound in earthy and sandy particles are usually of a darker colour, and of a softer substance.

In medical properties Galbanum strongly resembles Assafœtida, but is less powerful in its operation; it is expectorant and emmenagogue, and may be used, under similar circumstances, where the exhibition of Assafœtida is, from its offensive odour, objectionable. As an expectorant, it may be given in doses from gr. x. to ½oz in combination with ipecacuanha and any narcotic, two or three times a-day.

ASSAFŒTIDA OR GIANT FENNEL

Ferula persica

Class and Order, Pentandria Digynia. Nat. Ord. Umbelliferæ.
Gen. Char. *Fruit* compressed, flat, thickened at the edge, with three obtuse dorsal ribs, and banded intervals and jucture; *Flowers* polygamous; *Involucre* various.

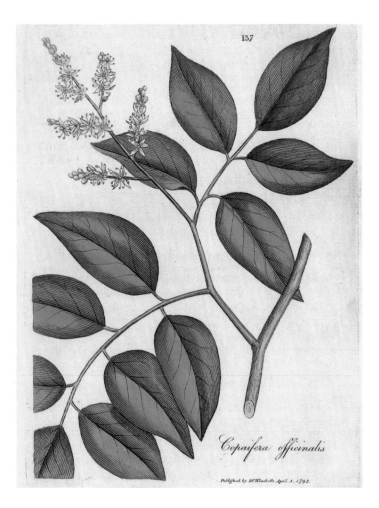

Copaifera officinalis

Published by Dr Woodville April 1.1792.

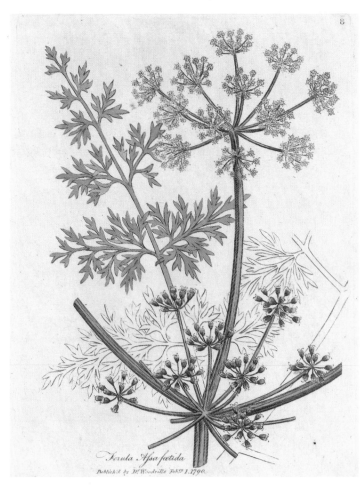

Ferula Assa fœtida

Published by Dr Woodville Feby 1.1790.

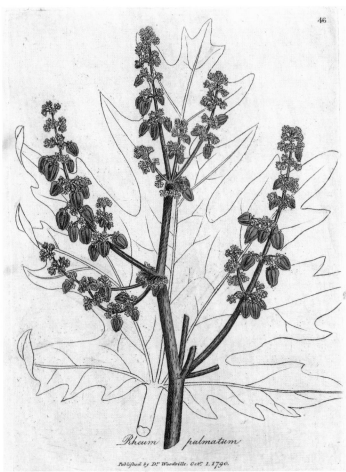

Rheum palmatum

Published by Dr Woodville Octr. 1.1790.

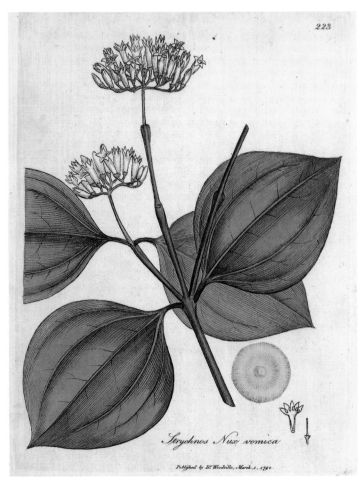

Strychnos Nux vomica

Published by Dr Woodville March 1.1794.

TOP LEFT: BALSAM OF COPAIVA OR COPAIBA, TOP RIGHT: ASSAFOETIDA OR GIANT FENNEL, BOTTOM LEFT: OFFICINAL OR PALMATED RHUBARB, BOTTOM RIGHT: NUX VOMICA OR POISON-NUT

THOUGH the present species yields the drug ASSAFŒTIDA, the one known as *F. assafœtida* has long been lost, but several of the species are supposed to yield a substance identical with the officinal drug; "which is procured by cutting across the top of the root, from whence its juices ooze out, and when dry it is scraped off as opium is from the capsule of the poppy. The plant grows three feet high, with yellow flowers, and hemlock-like leaves and habit; it is perennial, and is a native of Persia."—*Loudon.*

The drug is imported in irregular masses, composed of variously coloured clear, shining tears; it has a penetrating garlick-like odour, and a bitter acrid taste. Such samples as have the tears, of which the mass is formed, clear and white, with the bulk of the mass of a pale reddish brown, are to be preferred.

Assafœtida is the most powerful of the fœtid gums; it is stimulant, antispasmodic, expectorant, emmenagogue, and anthelmintic. From its stimulant nature, it must not be exhibited when inflammatory symptoms are present; it has been found useful in chronic catarrhs and asthmatic affection of worn-out habits. The best form of administering it as an expectorant is that of pill, combined with ipecacuanha and extract of conium; the dose is from four to twelve grains of the gum resin; to be repeated at short intervals.

GUM AMMONIACUM PLANT

Dorema ammoniacum

Class and Order, PENTANDRIA DIGYNIA. NAT. ORD. UMBELLIFERÆ.
Gen. Char. *Disk* epigynous, cup-shaped; *Carpels* compressed, marginate, three intermediate ridges filiform; *Interstices* with single *vittæ.*

ALTHOUGH the drug Ammoniacum has been known from the time of Dioscorides, the source from whence it has been obtained has remained in obscurity, and, as will be observed by the synonyms, has been referred to various plants of the family of *Umbelliferæ.* Recently the true plant has been discovered in the vicinity of Jezud Khart, a town of Irak El Ajam, the ancient Parthia, south of Ispahan. The plant is described by Mr. D. Don:

"Every part of the specimen is covered with drops of a gum possessing all the properties of *ammoniacum*; this circumstance alone, independent of any other evidence, would seem sufficient to remove all doubts on the subject. But, besides, I have carefully compared the specimen with the portions of inflorescence and fruit, which are found abundantly intermixed with the gum in the shops, and find them to agree in every particular. To avoid any confusion, and as the plant proves to be a new genus, I propose to call it DOREMA, from the Greek δόσημα, a gift of benefit; not that I consider the ammoniacum plant as pre-eminently deserving that title, but the name is at least a short one, and agreeable to the ear,—considerations not to be overlooked in nomenclature. The plant is perennial, and throws up from the root a cluster of leaves, and one or more strong, vigorous, naked stems, of three or four feet in height, divided into joints of five or six inches long, throwing out various branches of equal lengths. The white juice which forms the gum pervades the whole plant, but exudes chiefly from the principal stems. It either remains on them in lumps, or, falling to the ground, is gathered by the villagers in autumn, and is sold by them. The Ooshāk plant is to be met with no where but in the province of Irak, growing in very dry plains, gravelly soils, and exposed to an ardent sun."

The drug is imported in large irregular masses of an olive yellow colour, but whitish within; is tenacious, but breaks with a vitreous fracture; its odour is faint, and of a bitter pungent taste. It abounds in impurities, as seeds, pieces of stalks, leaves, and a variety of extraneous substances.

Ammoniacum is a stimulant, and is sometimes used as an antispasmodic and expectorant in asthmatic affections; it is usually combined with squill, assafœtida, or sedatives; it may also be administered in conjuction with ammonia.

GLOSSARY OF MEDICAL TERMS

Anasarca .... A disease similar to dropsy

Anodyne .... Relieving pain

Antiphlogistic .... Anti-inflammatory

Carminative .... A medicine that expels flatulence

Casting .... Vomiting

Cataplasm .... Poultice

Cathartic .... A purgative medicine

Decoction .... A medicine produced by boiling
roots, bark etc. in water

Demulcent .... A soothing medicine

Diaphoretic .... Inducing sweating

Diluent .... Increasing proportion of water in the blood

Diuretic .... Increasing flow of urine

Dropsy .... A disease in which watery fluid collects
in the body

Emetic .... Causing vomiting

Emmenagogue ...... Promoting menstruation

Epigastrium .... Part of the abdomen immediately over the
stomach

Febrifuge .... A medicine which reduces fever

Hydrothorax .... Water on the lungs

Icthyosis .... A skin disease that causes a scaly, harsh skin rash

Matrix .... Womb

Phrenitis .... Delirium

Poultice .... A soft heated mass of bread or
kaolin etc. applied to an inflamed or sore
area of skin

Rubefacient .... Counter-irritant

Scrofula .... Constitutional condition with glandular
swellings and a tendency to tuberculosis;
also called King's-evil

Strangury .... Painful urination drop by drop

Sudorific .... Inducing sweating

INDEX